THE MIRACLE OF
GARLIC

Practical Tips for
HEALTH AND HOME

DR PENNY STANWAY

WATKINS PUBLISHING

LONDON

This edition first published in the UK and USA 2013 by
Watkins Publishing Limited,
Sixth Floor, 75 Wells Street, London W1T 3QH

A member of Osprey Group

3 5 7 9 10 8 6 4 2

Designed and typeset by Jerry Goldie Graphic Design

Printed and bound in Italy by L.E.G.O.

A CIP record for this book is available from the British Library

ISBN: 978-1-78028-499-6

www.watkinspublishing.co.uk

Distributed in the USA and Canada by Sterling Publishing Co., Inc.
387 Park Avenue South, New York, NY 10016-8810

For information about custom editions, special sales, premium and
corporate purchases, please contact Sterling Special Sales
Department at 800-805-5489 or specialsales@sterlingpub.com

Contents

Introduction

Garlic is valued around the world as a flavouring ingredient, a food and a medicine. It belongs to the Alliaceae family, whose 750 species include onions, shallots, chives, leeks and ornamental alliums. The word 'garlic' originates from the Old English for 'spear' (*gar*) and 'leek' (*leac*). Its botanical name, *Allium sativum*, comes from the Greek for 'avoid' (presumably because of its smell) and 'cultivated'. In English alone its many other names include 'prince of herbs', 'food of love', 'nectar of the gods', 'devil's posy', 'camphor of the poor', 'poor man's treacle' ('treacle' from the Latin *theriaca*, meaning 'antidote to poison' or 'heal all'), 'onion stinker' and 'stinking Jenny/lily/rose'.

Today's garlic originated as a wild form in Central Asia more than 10,000 years ago. Over the centuries, this was cultivated and traded along the spice and silk routes to China, the Middle East and the Mediterranean. Eventually it reached Africa, Europe, Australia and the Americas. Today, China produces more than 12 million tonnes (metric tons) a year, which is three-quarters of the global crop. Other top producers, in order of harvest-size, include India, South Korea, Egypt, Russia, the US (especially California), Spain, Argentina, Burma and Ukraine.

Garlic's flavour is variously described as pungent, tangy, full, nutty, sweet and musky. It's an important ingredient in many dishes around the world. In Korea and China, the average traditional diet contains 8–12 cloves a day, while average consumption in the US is half to one clove a day. Some people, though, dislike its flavour as well as the scent that emanates from garlic eaters.

From the time of Ancient Egypt, around 4000BC, to the end of the 19th century, garlic was the most widely used medicinal plant in the world. It remains a popular traditional remedy for many ailments today. Garlic supplements are among the top-selling herbal supplements in the Western world, and thousands of scientific studies have investigated how garlic can promote good health.

Historically, garlic was also used in the art world: during the 13th–17th centuries, gilders used its sticky juice to attach gilding to picture frames and furniture. Nowadays, it is used in industry, too. Garlic oil (isolated by distilling garlic cloves with water) is in big demand because it contains compounds needed for the production of industrial chemicals called alkenes. Alkenes are used for making high-end lubricants, sealants for the glass industry, and binders used in solid propellants for rockets, as well as in the vulcanization of rubber.

Over the millennia, magical powers have been attributed to garlic, and it has been said to protect against vampires, werewolves, witches, sorcerers, demons and evil spirits! Even today some Greek midwives lay garlic in the delivery room to avert the 'evil eye' from the newborn baby, and in some countries people hang garlic outside their home to protect their family.

CHAPTER 1

Garlic Plants

Garlic is a perennial plant with a white, pink, brown or purple-striped bulb called a head. Its bulb is 4–7.5cm/1½–3in wide and has 4–25 parts called cloves. Each clove is made of two modified leaves – one forming its body, the other its papery wrappings (peel or skin). If you plant a mature clove, it develops into a new garlic plant.

Hardneck Garlic Plants (*Allium sativum ophioscorodon,* ophios or serpent garlics)

These plants are called bolters or top-setters because in the summer they produce a thick flower-stalk (scape), the leading end of which bears a papery capsule (topset or umbel) topped with a long point (beak). The stalk may loop or coil up to three times, making it look amazing in a flower arrangement. As it matures, it hardens and straightens. Within the capsule develops a cluster of up to several hundred tiny greenish, pink, red or purple flowers that rarely produce seeds. Among these are clove-like bulbils, numbering from a few to more than a hundred, depending on the variety. If you plant a mature bulbil, it develops into a new garlic plant.

The cloves are larger and easier to peel than those of softneck plants, and are often particularly well flavoured. They are, however, less numerous and cannot be stored for as long.

Varieties include:

- Rocamboles – 6–11 cloves with a rich, deep, sweetish flavour. These are many people's favourite and are excellent raw. They dislike wet soil. They have a thin brownish bulb wrapper that peels easily. They are the shortest-storing garlic (often only 3–6 months, or 6–8 if well grown and dried).

- Porcelains (Spanish garlic) – 4–6 large cloves with a hot, rich, musky flavour. Their 'heat' is due to a particularly high yield of allicin. They are the hardiest for cool climates, have a thick white bulb wrapper and are the second-longest storing after Silverskins (see page 3).

- Purple Stripe – 8–12 purple-striped cloves with a rich flavour. These are arguably the best garlic for roasting.

- Marbled Purple-Stripe – as for Purple Stripe.

- Glazed Purple-Stripe – as for Purple Stripe.

- Asiatics – bolt only weakly in warmer climates. They have a good flavour and are medium- to long-storing.

Softneck Garlic Plants (*Allium sativum sativum*, non-topsetters or non-bolters)

These plants produce a stalk that is only ever semi-stiff, and which softens and bends when the bulb is mature. There are no flowers. There may be a few bulbils above or even inside the bulb.

The cloves tend to be more numerous than those of hardneck

plants; they are also longer-storing, smaller and harder to peel.

Varieties include:

- Artichokes – 12–18 cloves with a fairly mild flavour. They can be stored for 6–9 months, are earlier-maturing than Silverskins and are the most common supermarket garlic in the US.

- Silverskins (Italians or Egyptians) – up to 24 cloves with a hot flavour. They are later-maturing than Artichokes and are the longest-storing garlics (often 6–12 months). Their soft stalks plait (braid) well, so are useful for making decorations.

- Creoles (Americans) – a rich, sweetish flavour that can be medium-hot. Their bulb wrappers may be red or purple. Sometimes they bolt and become hardnecks. They are long-storing and are the earliest-maturing garlics.

- Turbans – as for Creoles.

Hundreds of named strains of these varieties are grown worldwide. Besides varying in the number and size of their cloves, and in their storability, they also vary in the proportions and amounts of alliin (see page 10) they contain and therefore in their potential to produce allicin and allicin derivatives. This, in turn, affects their pungency, or heat.

Connoisseurs recommend thinking of garlic as we do wine, trying different varieties or strains to savour their different flavours. However, supermarkets tend to sell only softneck bulbs because their cloves can be planted mechanically, the plants need less care and the bulbs are longer-storing and therefore cheaper. So if you want to try hardneck varieties, you'll probably have to buy from a farmers' market or grow your own.

Spring Garlic (garlic shoots, or garlic scallions)

This is a very young garlic plant that, like a spring onion (scallion), is harvested whole in late spring before its bulb has swollen. It is sold in bunches and the whole plant is edible.

Green Garlic (young wet garlic)

This is a young garlic plant that is harvested whole in early summer when its bulb is small, its cloves have just separated and the above-ground parts are no more than 30cm/12in tall; any taller and the leaves would be tough to eat. Green garlic looks like a baby leek and needs no curing (see page 8). It is sold in bunches and the whole plant is edible.

Garlic Greens

These are the stalks of a garlic plant, harvested in early summer, leaving the bulb in the ground. The bulb then produces more stalks. Repeated harvesting and regrowth of garlic greens enables several crops to be enjoyed.

Many growers cut the stalks to increase the size of a plant's bulb. The stalks of a hardneck plant must be harvested before they straighten and harden.

Garlic-scented Plants

The elephant garlic plant (*Allium ampeloprasum*, or giant, great-headed, Tahitian or Russian garlic) is actually a wild leek. Its bulb weighs up to 450g/1lb and contains very large, yellowish, very mildly flavoured cloves. *Tulbaghia violacea* (society garlic) is another garlic-scented plant.

Wild garlics include *Allium canadense* (Canada garlic, field garlic, meadow leek, rose leek), *Allium oleraceum* (field garlic), *Alliaria petiolata* (garlic mustard, Jack-by-the-hedge), *Allium tricoccum* (buckrams, ramps or ramsons – so called because it smells as strongly as a ram), *Allium ursinum* (bear's garlic, bear's leek, broad-leaved garlic, wood garlic, Londoner's lily, stinking nanny, stink bombs), *Allium moly* (lily leek, sorcerer's garlic or, because of its large yellow flowers, golden garlic) and *Allium vineale* (crow garlic, wild onion). It is said that bear's garlic or leek was so called because bears like digging up its bulbs. Wild garlic has a stronger scent and flavour than true garlic. Some people cook it, for example, stir-fried with nettles and sorrel. Cows that graze on wild garlic produce garlic-scented milk; lambs that eat it have garlicky meat; and if it grows among wheat, barley, oats or rye, its bulbils give the grain a garlic taint.

Growing Your Own

Start with cloves (from a home-grown or shop-bought bulb) or bulbils (from a home-grown plant, or a seed supplier – who may call them seeds or seed garlic). Avoid cloves from bulbs sold as food, though, as they may have been irradiated (see page 43) and so will not sprout. Follow the tips given below, which come from professional growers.

Bulbils have four advantages:

• Different varieties are available from seed suppliers.

• There is no risk of soil-borne disease.

• Hardnecks produce many more bulbils than cloves.

• Plants from bulbils often do better than their parents.

However, planting bulbils may produce a single-cloved bulb (a round). And while this will grow larger each year if left in the ground, some varieties take two or three years to form fully separated cloves.

Preparing the soil

Enrich and lighten the soil if necessary, as garlic prefers rich, light, loose, well-drained, sandy or gravelly soil with a moderate amount of humus (organic matter) and a neutral to slightly acidic pH (acidity index). Grow garlic in a raised bed if your soil is poorly drained. In colder climates, plant cloves or bulbils at the beginning of autumn (the fall).

Choosing varieties

Porcelains and Purple Stripes are particularly successful in areas with cold winters, Artichokes and Creoles in areas with warm winters.

Planting

Plant cloves with their tips uppermost. Plant larger bulbils so the end that was attached to the plant points down; it doesn't matter which way you plant tiny bulbils. Cover cloves and bulbils with 1.25–10cm/½–4in soil (the colder the expected winter, the more covering they need). Space them 10–18cm/4–7in apart, with 25cm/10in between rows.

In very cold areas, plant cloves in a seed tray of multi-purpose compost in a cold frame or cool greenhouse, and plant out in spring.

Cloves or bulbils can be planted in a 4.5–9 litre/1–2 gallon container if protected from freezing in very cold weather.

Consider growing garlic on a sunny indoor windowsill.

Mulching and cloches
In cold areas, mulch in winter and cover with cloches in frosty weather.

Fertilizing
Give foliar feeds.

Watering
Water well in dry weather so the cloves swell.

Weeding
Keep weeds down, as garlic is easily overwhelmed.

Cutting stalks
If intending to harvest a hardneck's bulb, help its cloves swell by cutting off its stalk while it's still looped, which is about 3 weeks before the bulb is ready. Some garlic-growers report that leaving the stalk on reduces bulb size by a third.

Harvesting
Harvest the bulb when only the top 5–6 leaves remain green. If you intend to harvest a hardneck's bulbils for planting, don't harvest the bulb when you normally would. Instead, wait for the bulbils to mature, then harvest them, and only then harvest the bulb. Hardneck

bulbs harvested this late store for only about 2 months, softnecks 3–4 months, but you can eat them straight away or plant their cloves.

Drying (curing)
Spread the harvested plants on newspaper or tie them into bundles and hang them with their bulbs hanging downwards, somewhere undercover, shaded, well-ventilated and frost-free. Handle the bulbs gently so they do not bruise. Let the bulbs dry for 2–6 weeks or until all their leaves are brown.

Tidying up the bulbs
Cut off the stalks, leaving a neck of 2.5cm/1in on hardnecks, less on softnecks. Trim the roots to half that length, brush soil from the trimmed roots, and remove soil-stained outer wrappers.

Companion Planting

Garlic plants help to repel pests from certain other plants. Roses, for example, are said to be more resistant to the fungal infection blackspot if planted near garlic. They are also said to smell sweeter. Other plants said to benefit from garlic as a neighbour include beans, beetroot, cabbages, carrots, cucumbers, lettuces, peas, potatoes, strawberries and tomatoes. Trials that have sited garlic alongside sugar beet or winter wheat have had encouraging results.

Scientists report that a garlic product (ECOguard, see page 128) is one of the most effective pesticides for slugs and snails. They also claim it is worth spraying soil with water containing crushed garlic cloves.

CHAPTER 2

What's in Garlic

There are two special things about garlic. First, more than 160 of a garlic bulb's constituents are bioactive, meaning they can affect our body. The amounts are tiny, but can nevertheless contribute to health, especially if consumed regularly. Second, garlic's odour, flavour and tingle on the tongue are unique.

Here we'll consider garlic's contents, odour and flavour, as well as what's in garlic supplements, and the reasons for the recommendations in Chapter 3 on storing, preparing and cooking garlic. Go directly to the next chapter if you prefer to skip the science.

The constituents most important to our health and our enjoyment of garlic are its sulfur compounds.

Sulfur Compounds

Compared weight for weight with onions, garlic is four times richer in sulfur-containing compounds. These include certain enzymes (such as glutathione) and amino acids (cysteine, cystine, methionine, taurine), as well as various cysteine derivatives. All these bioactive compounds are vital for our metabolism and can be obtained from various foods. But it is the uniquely high content of cysteine derivatives that is largely responsible for garlic's scent, flavour and health-giving potential.

Cysteine derivatives

Fresh whole raw garlic cloves contain three groups of these water-soluble, odour-free sulfur compounds:

- Alliin and other cysteine sulfoxides. The amount of alliin (pronounced 'alley-in'), for example, varies ten-fold, depending on the variety of bulb and the soil and climate in which it grew.

- Gamma-glutamyl cysteines. Storing garlic at a cool temperature slowly converts these into S-cysteines (see below).

- S-cysteines. S-allyl cysteine, for example, is arguably garlic's most important sulfur compound.

Alliinase

Crushing, chopping or chewing raw garlic cloves sparks a cascade of activity by tearing open tiny compartments containing the enzyme alliinase. This exposes it to oxygen and water, enabling it to convert alliin into sulfenic acid. The more a clove is damaged, the more sulfenic acid is produced. Within a few seconds, sulfenic acid forms allicin and other pungent thiosulfinates. This time lag explains why, if you chew raw garlic, several seconds elapse before it tastes pungent. The sulfenic acid and allicin in newly crushed garlic can inflame or burn the cells of our skin, mouth, throat, stomach and eyes. Garlic produces these substances to deter invasion by soil fungi, bacteria and parasites.

Allicin production is steady for 6¼ minutes, then spurts for

½ minute. This cycle repeats every 6¾ minutes until 90 minutes, which is when the allicin level peaks. This has implications for cooks. *The longer you wait up to 90 minutes before using newly crushed or chopped garlic, the more allicin is formed.* Wait 7 minutes and you benefit from the first cycle. Wait 14 minutes, and you also benefit from the second. Wait 90 minutes, and you get the maximum yield.

However, alliinase is permanently deactivated (preventing the conversion of alliin to allicin) if crushed or chopped garlic is:

- cooked – because heat (depending on its degree and the cooking time) destroys alliinase;

- mixed with lemon juice or vinegar – because acids of pH 3 or below destroy alliinase; or

- eaten – because normal stomach acidity and body heat break down almost all the alliinase in swallowed garlic, leading to a 99 per cent loss of potential allicin production. Normal stomach juice has a pH from 1 (highly acid – for example, while eating a low-protein meal) to 5 (low acid – for example, on waking). If you have low stomach acid (for example, because of ageing, stress, antacid or acid-suppressant medication, or a diet low in vegetables), or if you dilute it by drinking water, or if you take an enteric-coated garlic supplement, more alliinase may get through the stomach. But most will then be inactivated by your intestinal juice and cells.

So the sooner you cook newly crushed or chopped garlic, mix it with something acidic, or eat it, the more alliin is retained and the less allicin is produced. Conversely, the longer you leave crushed or chopped garlic before you cook it, mix it with something acidic or eat it, the less alliin is retained and the more allicin is produced.

Alliin and allicin (and, most importantly, allicin's derivatives) each have a particular range of health benefits (see page 14). If you want garlic to contain relatively more alliin or allicin, leave crushed or chopped garlic for less or more time within the 90-minute timeframe, respectively.

Allicin is unstable and eventually converted by enzymes into oil-soluble allicin derivatives (see page 13). If you leave crushed or chopped garlic at a warm room temperature of 23°C/73°F, half its allicin is converted within 2½ days, the rest over a longer time. Its conversion takes longer in a cooler room.

Allicin's conversion to its derivatives is *faster* if crushed or chopped garlic is:

- cooked – for example, 45 minutes of oven-roasting, or 1 minute of microwaving, converts all its allicin;

- mixed with vegetable oil – this converts half the allicin within 3 hours; also it converts relatively more into ajoene and vinyl dithiins than into allyl sulfides (see page 13); or

- mixed with warm water at 37°C/99°F – this converts half the allicin within 24 hours.

In addition, allicin's conversion is *slower* if crushed or chopped garlic is:

- mixed with room-temperature or cool water – this converts half the allicin within 12 days at 23°C/73°F, 32 days at 15°C/59°F, 1 year at 4°C/39°F;

- mixed with alcohol – this converts half the allicin within 12 days;

- refrigerated – this slows allicin conversion 20-fold, so half might, for example, be converted within 60 days; or

- mixed with vinegar, lemon juice or wine: this converts all the
  allicin over 2 years.

Allicin derivatives include allyl sulfides (such as diallyl disulfide,
diallyl trisulfide, allyl methyl sulfide), allyl mercaptan, methyl
mercaptan, ajoene (pronounced 'ah-ho-een'; a disulfide) and vinyl
dithiins (pronounced 'die-thigh-ins'). Their bioactivity and stability
account for most of the health benefits previously attributed to
allicin. They remain stable for a year or so at room temperature, or
longer if refrigerated. Diallyl disulfide, ajoene and vinyl dithiins are
the most stable.

What happens to garlic in the body

When you consume garlic, its water-soluble and oil-soluble
compounds affect the body in different ways.

- Garlic's water-soluble compounds (such as alliin, gamma-
  glutamyl cysteine and S-allyl cysteine) have small molecules
  that easily diffuse from the intestine into the capillaries (tiny
  blood vessels) in the intestinal wall. These capillaries empty into
  the hepatic portal vein which takes blood directly to the liver.
  Gamma-glutamyl cysteine is converted into S-allyl cysteine,
  which contributes heavily to garlic's health benefits and can be
  measured in the blood, liver and urine. The liver converts alliin
  into diallyl disulfide, which is subsequently converted into allyl
  mercaptan. Interestingly, the liver's cytochrome P-450 enzyme
  can convert dialllyl disulfide back into allicin.

- Garlic's oil-soluble compounds (allicin and allicin derivatives)
  have large molecules, so only very small amounts can diffuse

from the intestine into the capillaries. Any allicin that enters the blood quickly reacts with substances such as the enzyme glutathione peroxidase, or breaks down into allicin derivatives, or enters cells.

However, the large molecules can diffuse into the lymph vessels in the intestinal wall, because the pressure in these vessels is very low. They then travel in lymph, where they may escape into cells, be used or broken down, or be emptied into the blood in the subclavian veins. When allyl sulfides, ajoene and vinyl dithiins reach the liver, they are either used or broken down into substances such as allyl methyl sulfide and allyl mercaptan.

What happens to garlic on the skin

When garlic is applied to the skin, some of its sulfur compounds penetrate it and enter the blood. So if garlic is rubbed on to the soles of the feet, for example, the person's breath is scented with garlic within 10 minutes or so.

Health-promoting effects of garlic's sulfur compounds

Scientists believe that alliin, gamma-glutamyl cysteine, S-allyl cysteine and allicin derivates such as allyl sulfides, ajoene and vinyl dithiins account for most of garlic's health-promoting effects. Studies indicate that these and certain other sulfur compounds have various actions:

- Anti-cancer – test-tube studies show that S-allyl cysteine inhibits growth of prostate- and breast-cancer cells; S-allyl mercaptocysteine reduces cancer-cell multiplication; and certain sulfur compounds discourage the cancer-promoting effects of acrylamide (in cooked carbohydrates) and heterocyclic amines (in cooked meat). Alliin, S-allyl cysteine, allicin, diallyl disulfide, ajoene, vinyl dithiins, thiacremonone, allixin, sulfur amino acids, glutathione and sulforaphane (produced from glutathione when garlic is chopped or crushed) have antioxidant and possibly anti-cancer activity. Diallyl disulfide and diallyl trisulfide discourage the spread of cancer cells in lymph. Diallyl trisulfide discourages the spread of lung-cancer cells.

- Anti-clotting – allicin, ajoene, vinyl dithiins and diallyl disulfide are powerful anti-clotting agents in the test tube. Ajoene has equal potency to aspirin, but without its possible side effects.

- Anti-diabetic – allicin and allyl propyl disulfide may protect insulin by locking on to it so insulin-inactivating compounds found in people with diabetes can't work. Early studies suggest that sulforaphane has anti-diabetic properties.

- Anti-microbial – vapour from crushed garlic can kill certain bacteria up to 20cm/8in away. Test-tube studies show that crushed garlic and certain garlic supplements inhibit the growth of certain bacteria, increase our natural killer cells' anti-viral activity, and reduce the 'stickability' of fungi by altering the fat content of their cell membranes. Allicin acts against a wide range of bacteria and can break up biofilms (sheets of bacteria with high resistance to antibiotics and our immune-system's defences; present in an estimated four in five infections). Bacteria don't become resistant to allicin because, unlike many antibiotics, allicin penetrates them and inactivates their cysteine-protease enzymes. Allicin also acts against certain viruses, fungi and protozoa. It has been patented in the US for its antibiotic and anti-fungal effects. Various sulfides have anti-bacterial, anti-viral and anti-fungal actions; ajoenes have the highest anti-viral activity. Sulforaphane and allixin have anti-microbial action.

- Anti-obesity – laboratory studies suggest that allyl-sulfides discourage obesity by increasing adrenaline and noradrenaline, hormones that stimulate trialglycerol metabolism and are thought to boost heat production in brown fat (very metabolically active fat between the shoulder-blades). Ajoene can inactivate gastric lipase (an enzyme needed for fat digestion). And vinyl dithiins may discourage pro-inflammatory conditions that promote obesity.

- Antioxidant and anti-inflammatory – alliin, S-allyl cysteine, sulfenic acid, allicin, allyl disulfide, diallyl disulfide, ajoene, vinyl dithiins, allyl mercaptan, thiacremonone, sulfur amino acids, sulforaphane and glutathione have these effects in the test tube. Red blood cells convert diallyl disulfide and diallyl trisulfide to hydrogen sulfide, which increases certain anti-inflammatory factors (NFκB p65, Nrf2 and GLUT 4 and PPAR delta).

- Smooth-muscle-relaxing – laboratory studies show that gamma-glutamyl cysteine acts like the ACE (angiotensin-converting enzyme) -inhibitor drugs used for high blood pressure, heart failure and strokes. Hydrogen sulfide (see above) expands arteries, which lowers blood pressure. Certain compounds stimulate the release of prostaglandins that relax smooth muscle and therefore expand arteries.

- Cholesterol-lowering – laboratory studies indicate that S-allyl cysteine reduces cholesterol production via a statin-like action (statins being cholesterol-reducing drugs). Gamma-glutamyl cysteine, diallyl disulfide, diallyltrisulfide, allyl mercaptan and vinyl dithiins may also have cholesterol-lowering action. And ajoene reduces cholesterol production. However, claims that garlic lowers cholesterol in people remain controversial.

- Detoxifying – sulfates detoxify substances such as paracetamol (acetaminophen), estrogen and adrenaline by a process called sulfation. Allyl sulfides are potent detoxifiers. Glutathione can detoxify several potentially dangerous substances, including paracetamol. And sulforaphane can detoxify certain carcinogens and toxins. Garlic's sulfur compounds can also help to remove heavy metals such as arsenic, lead and mercury from the body.

- Digestive-juice-stimulating – garlic encourages normal stomach contractions and promotes the flow of stomach juice.

- Immunity-enhancing – our immune system uses diallyl disulfide to make antibodies. And test-tube studies indicate that garlic can boost the performance of natural killer cells – white cells that help to destroy cancer cells and virus-infected cells.

Other Constituents of Garlic

Besides sulfur compounds, garlic cloves contain water (which accounts for over half their weight), proteins, free amino acids, oils, fats, carbohydrates, vitamins, other minerals and other constituents.

Proteins and amino acids

The proteins include certain enzymes (such as alliinase, peroxidase and myrosinase) and lectins (sugar-binding proteins that are currently being investigated for their anti-cancer potential).

The 17 free amino acids in garlic include arginine (an antioxidant that helps to maintain healthy blood pressure and is being studied for anti-cancer potential) and four sulfur-containing amino acids: cysteine, cystine, methionine and taurine (essential for our body's structural proteins, including keratin in nails and hair, and collagen in joints).

Oils and fats

Garlic's essential oil, found mainly in its cell membranes, consists of free fatty acids, fats called glycolipids and phospholipids, and terpenes. In cut, chopped or crushed garlic, these are joined by oil-soluble allicin and allicin derivatives.

Carbohydrates

These include:

- Mucilage – a sticky substance that forms nearly half a clove's weight.

- Sugars – 17 sorts, including glucose, oligosaccharides, fructose and fructans, which may enhance our immunity (fermentation of fructans by bowel bacteria discourages gastro-enteritis, constipation and, perhaps, high blood pressure, high cholesterol and cancer.

- Pectin – found in garlic cloves' papery skins and extracted for commercial use

Vitamins

Garlic's main vitamins are B6 and C; others include A, B1, B2, B3, biotin (B7) and E. The S-allyl group common to many of garlic's sulfur compounds aids absorption of vitamin B1.

Minerals

Garlic is rich in phosphorus, potassium, selenium, sulfur and the trace elements germanium and manganese.

Garlic is the richest in selenium of all vegetables. Interestingly, it can extract selenium even when the concentration of this mineral in soil is poor. While a large clove contains only 1.6 per cent of the US Recommended Dietary Allowance (RDA) for selenium, a large clove grown in selenium-enriched soil can contain four times this RDA. Garlic's sulfur content enhances the antioxidant power of its selenium.

Garlic is the richest in sulfur of all vegetables, containing at least four times as much as onions and cabbage, for example.

Our body's sulfur is distributed among certain enzymes and bile acids, as well as insulin, biotin, collagen, elastin, proteogly-cans ('mucopolysaccharides', in connective tissues and joint fluid), coenzyme A, lipoic acid and the antioxidant enzyme glutathione.

Studies suggest that the average diet in the US, for example, lacks sufficient sulfur. Deficiency often goes undetected as it causes no clearly defined symptoms. So the average person might do well to eat more sulfur-rich foods. Meat, fish and eggs are the richest sources, followed by pulses, but garlic is useful, too, even though the amounts are small.

Other

Garlic also includes:

• Flavonoids – including myricetin and apignin (being investigated for its anti-cancer effects). Many, notably quercetin, allixin and anthocyanins, are powerful antioxidants. Quercetin also has anti-histamine and anti-viral properties, can lower blood sugar by stimulating insulin production, and can strengthen capillaries. Allixin helps to prevent the formation of prostaglandins that encourage inflammation, blood clotting and cancer growth; it also has anti-microbial effects and enhances nerve growth.

- Anthocyanins – flavonoid derivatives and phenolic compounds that include caffeic acid, ferulic acid and tannins (which have antioxidant properties).

- Terpenes – odoriferous compounds in garlic's oil, including citral (lemon-scented), geraniol (rose-scented), linalool (with a sweet, woody, lavender scent) and phellandrenes (with a peppery, minty or citrus scent).

- Plant hormones – for example, glucokinin ('plant insulin'), which is thought to lower blood sugar and so protect the pancreas from exhausting itself by having to produce a large amount of insulin.

- Saponins – steroid-like substances thought to have cholesterol- and blood-pressure-lowering actions and to encourage healthy proportions of micro-organisms in the bowel. They are also thought to help protect against bowel cancer by breaking down the cholesterol-rich membranes of its cells. Certain saponins have anti-inflammatory, anti-microbial and anti-parasitic activities.

Garlic's Odour and Flavour

These arise mainly from volatile oil-soluble thiosulfinates such as allicin (which has a slightly sweet and piquant garlicky scent, and makes the tongue tingle) and its derivatives (such as diallyl disulfide, allyl methyl disulfide, allyl mercaptan and methyl mercaptan). They also come from certain water-soluble substances, including alliin, methiin and other cysteine sulfoxides. The scents of garlic's terpenes (see page 20) add to the complexity of its odour and flavour.

Differences in the variety of garlic, the climatic conditions, the soil's sulfur content and how garlic is stored account for variations in odour and flavour. Garlic and onion smell and taste different mainly because they contain differing amounts of cysteine sulfoxides; for example, there is more isoalliin in onions, and more alliin in garlic.

The absence of garlic odour in dishes containing garlic implies they contain little in the way of volatile oil-soluble sulfur compounds, probably because crushed garlic was used before its alliinase could release allicin.

Garlic breath

Chewing and swallowing garlic releases sulfur compounds that immediately scent saliva, and mucus in the throat. This scents breath with garlic's 'primary odour'.

Certain sulfur compounds, including allyl methyl sulfide, are excreted from the lungs and in sweat for several hours after eating garlic. This scents breath and sweat with garlic's 'secondary odour'.

Sulfur compounds can also scent other body fluids, including urine and breast milk. Interestingly, babies spend longer breastfeeding (nursing) when their mothers have eaten garlic, implying they like the taste.

Our nose is so sensitive to the scent of garlic's volatile sulfur compounds on the breath that it can detect less than one part in a billion. However, the nose's olfactory sensors soon tire of the scent on another person's breath, especially if you have eaten garlic yourself.

See page 41 for suggestions on dealing with garlic breath.

Garlic Supplements

The four main commercially produced garlic supplements are garlic powder, aged garlic extract, garlic oil and garlic oil-macerate. They are available in pharmacies, online and in certain supermarkets and health-food shops.

Which you choose (see page 85) will depend on the health benefits you are seeking, since different production methods result in different ranges and levels of bioactive compounds. While the composition of garlic powder is closer to that of raw garlic than any other supplement, garlic powder may nevertheless contain less than half the allicin present in the equivalent amount of fresh garlic.

The amounts and potency of the compounds in garlic supplements often remain unclear. Also, the amounts of a particular compound in different brands of a particular type of supplement can be very different. In addition, some products are not standardized for any particular bioactive compound, so you cannot be sure how much of that compound they contain.

Some manufacturers add herbs such as mistletoe or hawthorn to their garlic supplements. Some add parsley in the probably forlorn hope that it will overcome secondary garlic odour, and others add other substances, such as cayenne (to expand arteries) and selenium or vitamins (hoping this might help to prevent or fight cancer).

Lastly, pure allicin is available in various formulations.

Garlic powder

Commercially produced garlic-powder supplements usually come as capsules, but are also available as tablets or ointment.

Garlic powder is made by slicing, drying and grinding fresh raw garlic cloves. It takes 1–1.2kg/2lb 4oz–2lb 6oz to produce 450g/1lb garlic powder.

The range of constituents in a well-produced garlic-powder supplement is as in whole raw garlic. But the processing can alter their amounts and proportions.

The alliinase in cloves remains safe but temporarily inactive (because of the lack of water), provided the temperature stays below 50–60°C/122–140°F. Rehydrating a garlic-powder supplement with water activates its alliinase, so it converts alliin to allicin. But alliinase is destroyed by normal stomach acidity. So if you particularly want allicin to be produced and to survive your stomach acid (so you can benefit from allicin and its derivatives), you need to do one of the following:

- Empty garlic powder from a capsule into a glass of water, stir and leave to stand: the longer you leave it, up to 90 minutes, the more allicin is produced. When you drink the garlic-powder-containing water, the water can dilute your stomach acid.

- Drink a glass of water to dilute your stomach acid, then swallow an enteric-coated product (see below).

Note that some manufacturers treat garlic powder with sulfur dioxide to reduce discoloration, and with hydrogen peroxide, salt solution or irradiation to eradicate bacterial contamination. These processes may alter the range and amounts of sulfur compounds.

Enteric-coated tablets

The majority of garlic-powder tablets are enteric-coated – meaning their manufactured 'shell' protects their contents from stomach acid. Historically, the expectation was that such a coating would dissolve only when the tablet reached the intestine, and that the garlic powder would then rehydrate so its alliinase could act on alliin to produce allicin. This gave rise to claims for a product's 'allicin potential'. But the reality is almost always different, because:

- too little alliinase may be present in the garlic powder;
- an enteric coating may dissolve early, allowing stomach acid to destroy the alliinase;
- an enteric coating may not dissolve in the intestine;
- intestinal juice inhibits allicin production by 40 per cent; and
- intestinal cells may break down allicin.

Test-tube experiments that mimic conditions in the stomach can predict allicin release, but few manufacturers provide such information. Also, this figure does not reflect what happens in real life: one study found that three in four types of enteric-coated product released less than 15 per cent of the expected amount of allicin.

Sometimes garlic powder or oil is put into gelatine capsules. However, stomach acid breaks down gelatine and prevents alliinase from converting alliin into allicin.

Garlic extracts

These are usually made by soaking whole or sliced garlic cloves in alcohol and water. The solution is then concentrated and can be dried, ground into a powder and formed into tablets.

Garlic extracts mainly contain water-soluble sulfur compounds, such as S-allyl cysteine and S-allyl mercaptocysteine. These two compounds are the least odorous of garlic's sulfur compounds. Garlic extracts may also contain allixin, S-1-propenyl cysteine and fructosyl arginine – a potent antioxidant not present in raw or cooked garlic.

Garlic extracts can be standardized according to their content of S-allyl cysteine.

Aged garlic extract is made by soaking garlic cloves in alcohol and water for up to 20 months. This allows the ongoing conversion of gamma-glutamyl cysteines to S-allyl cysteine and S-allyl mercapto-cysteine. Aged garlic extract is also rich in flavonoids such as allixin, and in fructosyl arginine. It also contains the antioxidant enzymes catylase and glutathione peroxidase.

However, it contain extremely little alliin, no active alliinase, little allicin, and only traces of allicin derivatives. Indeed, its total content of sulfur compounds is only one tenth of that of fresh or cooked garlic.

Manufacturers sometimes enrich aged garlic extract with other health-promoting compounds, such as vitamins B or E, co-enzyme Q, cayenne, hawthorn or fish oil or its acids (EPA and DHA), yeast, kelp, whey or digestive enzymes.

Steam-distilled garlic oil

This is the oldest type of commercial garlic supplement and is usually sold in capsules called perles. To produce garlic oil, steam is passed through crushed fresh raw garlic cloves, and the oil-rich steam condensed to form a reddish-brown oil.

Steam-distilled garlic oil differs in several ways from garlic's essential oil (see 'Ether-extracted garlic oil', page 26). It consists mainly of allicin-derived sulfides, many of which have a strong odour. In particular, it is rich in diallyl disulfide and diallyl trisulfide. While the amounts of these substances are vastly greater than in raw garlic or garlic powder, studies suggest that they are not as bioactive.

It takes about 450g/1lb garlic to produce 1g/just over ⅓₀oz steam-distilled oil. It is therefore very expensive. Supplement manufacturers usually sell it in capsules, perhaps diluted with a cheaper vegetable oil. The concentration of garlic oil in the average finished product is often as low as 1 per cent.

Ether-extracted garlic oil

Extracting garlic's oil with ether produces an oil that contains volatile oil-soluble sulfur compounds formed by the conversion of allicin and other thiosulfinates. Compared with steam-distilled garlic oil, this oil contains nine times as much of the vinyl dithiins and allyl sulfides and four times as much ajoene.

A medium (4g/just under ⅛oz) clove of fresh raw garlic produces only about 4mg of this oil.

Garlic oil-macerate

Garlic oil-macerate is made by chopping or crushing (macerating) garlic, mixing it with vegetable oil, then leaving the mixture for 24 hours at room temperature before straining out the pieces of garlic. The resulting garlic oil-macerate is put into capsules to create garlic perles.

During manufacture, some of the garlic's alliin is converted to allicin. This quickly converts into other sulfur compounds such as sulfides, ajoene and vinyl dithiins. Garlic oil-macerate is the only garlic supplement that contains significant amounts of ajoene and vinyl dithiins, and much of its bioactivity is thought to be due to the vinyl dithiins.

However, garlic oil-macerate contains much lower levels of

diallyl disulfide and diallyl trisulfide than does steam-distilled garlic oil.

Low-odour or odour-free garlic tablets or capsules

Enteric-coated products are 'low-odour' in that they prevent primary garlic breath but not the secondary sort.

Odour-free garlic is produced by preventing alliinase from working, so that allicin and its derivatives cannot be produced. This can be done by:

- exposing garlic to fumaric acid;

- physically separating alliinase from garlic;

- freeze-drying garlic mixed with cyclodextrin;

- heating garlic;

- producing garlic tablets without an enteric coating, so gastric acid destroys alliinase; or

- mixing crushed garlic with yeasts that break down allicin into non-smelly sulfur compounds.

However, such products mostly lack the health benefits of allicin and its derivatives.

Timed-release garlic tablets or capsules

These are created in a way that delays the release of their contents. The aim is for each dose to have a longer and steadier effect.

Allicin

Purified stablilized allicin is available as capsules, liquid and cream.

The suggested daily dose of powdered allicin in capsules is 3.6–5.4mg, which equates to the potential allicin yield from one medium clove of garlic.

Other garlic products

These include garlic syrup (see recipe on page 40), garlic tincture and garlic juice.

For information on which garlic supplement is best suited for which common ailment, see page 90.

CHAPTER 3

Choosing and Using Garlic

The tips in this chapter come from wisdom handed down over generations, the practical experience of growers and sellers, and observations from scientists.

Choosing a Bulb

When buying garlic, choose a bulb with firm plump cloves, dry wrappers and no hint of mould or discoloration. If a recipe needs a lot of garlic, choose a bulb with large cloves if possible, as they will be quicker to peel.

Using Garlic

Separate only the cloves you need.

Peeling

Fresh cloves are harder to peel. Make peeling easier by soaking cloves in water for an hour, or boiling them in water for 20 seconds.

Cut each clove above its base then peel off its wrapper with your fingertips or a knife. Alternatively, put a clove on a chopping board and press it with the flat surface of a broad sturdy knife blade to break its wrapper and make it easier to peel, or use a polyurethane garlic peeler (which looks like a piece of giant macaroni). Put it on a worktop and insert some cloves, then roll it backwards and forwards several times. Discard any cloves that look greyish or yellowish, or are dry and stringy inside.

Crushing or chopping

The smaller the pieces of garlic, the greater the damage, the larger the potential yield of allicin and the stronger the flavour. The longer you leave crushed or chopped garlic to stand (up to 90 minutes), the more allicin it yields (see page 10).

To crush a clove, choose one of the following options: chop it then squash the pieces with the flat surface of a broad sturdy knife blade; just squash it; use a garlic crusher; or use a pestle and mortar.

You don't have to peel a clove before crushing it, though many people find it easier to do so.

Soaking

Some people soak crushed or chopped garlic in milk, vinegar or alcohol, or boil cloves in water or milk, before use. This makes the flavour milder because sulfur compounds diffuse into the liquid. But you then lose the health benefits unless you consume the liquid too.

Sprouting

The green shoots of sprouting garlic can be bitter, but when chopped they make a good garnish for salads or a flavourful addition to stir-fries. If you prefer, cut a sprouted clove in half and discard the shoot.

Juicing

Some people add garlic juice when preparing vegetable juice, some use it to flavour food and others add it to water to make 'garlic water' for bathing skin infections or wounds (see page 41). One garlic bulb produces up to 4 tablespoons juice. To extract the juice, whizz peeled cloves in a blender until smooth. Spoon the purée into a fine sieve over a bowl and use a wooden spoon to force the juice through.

Cooking with Garlic

Leaving newly crushed or chopped garlic to stand for up to 90 minutes enables the production of allicin, which has a hot garlicky flavour. The longer you leave crushed or chopped garlic, up to 90 minutes, the more allicin is formed and so the 'hotter' and more garlicky the garlic will taste. Conversely, the sooner you use crushed or chopped garlic within that 90-minute timeframe, the milder and less garlicky it will taste.

Cooking crushed or chopped garlic destroys its alliinase, so no more alliin can be converted into allicin. Heat also encourages the allicin already produced to be converted into allicin derivatives, many of which also taste garlicky and add complexity to the flavour. Many of garlic's health benefits stem from its allicin derivatives. However, alliin has valuable health benefits, too, so it could be wise to conserve some by not waiting the full 90 minutes after crushing or chopping.

Just 60 seconds of microwaving or 45 minutes of oven-cooking newly crushed garlic destroy its alliinase.

Whole cloves do not produce allicin or allicin derivatives because they haven't been damaged. Cooking them for a long time at a relatively high temperature, for example, by roasting, deepens their flavour; it also sweetens them by creating a compound 50–70 times as sweet as table sugar, albeit in very small amounts.

Burning garlic gives it a nasty taste and destroys its antioxidants. Unfortunately, garlic burns quickly, so you need to pay close attention when frying it. Some people boil cloves in water for half a minute before frying them, as this prevents them tasting unpleasant if they do brown too much.

Careful frying produces a lovely rich nutty flavour. It also allows garlic's antioxidants to reduce heat-induced oxidation damage to frying oil and other foods. When frying:

- Use a heavy-based pan.

- Heat the oil before adding the garlic.

- Fry any onions first, and add the garlic when the onions are almost cooked.

- Add garlic last after any other foods too.

- Use only moderate heat, but make sure the garlic sizzles and turns golden (and therefore fries) and doesn't just steam and stay white.

- Keep stirring.

- Remove the pan from the heat when the garlic turns golden, but before it browns. Crushed garlic cooks in less than 1 minute, chopped garlic takes a little longer.

- Consider discarding garlic when it is cooked to golden, then stir-frying other foods in the garlic-flavoured oil.

When making stock, use unpeeled cloves because their wrappings are rich in quercetin. Before roasting garlic, snip the tips from cloves so it is easy to squeeze out their soft centres later.

Storing Garlic

Cool moist conditions encourage sprouting, while hot dry conditions make garlic bulbs dry out faster.

Commercial producers and distributors may store garlic at very cold temperatures of 0°C/32°F or lower to prevent sprouting. However, removal from this cold storage tends to stimulate sprouting within 2–4 weeks and can encourage rotting, whereas garlic that has not been cold-stored tends to keep longer. Keeping garlic at a temperature of 0-4°C/32-40°F, which is refrigerator temperature, encourages sprouting.

At home, garlic is best stored uncovered or loosely covered in a dark, dry place at 10–20°C/ 50–68°F and ideally at 13–14°C/56–58°F. This is because:

- This temperature discourages sprouting, rotting and drying-out.

- Good ventilation provides garlic with the oxygen its cells need to breathe, helping to keep them healthy and rot resistant. Options include a terracotta 'garlic-keeper' pot, or a net bag. Plastic and paper bags are unsuitable.

- Darkness helps to prevent drying or greening.

- Air humidity should be 40–60 per cent (ideally 45–50 per cent); any higher encourages rotting and root growth: any lower dries garlic faster. The easy-to-peel wrappers of hardneck-garlic cloves make them dessicate faster.

The temperature in a refrigerator encourages sprouting, and its humidity encourages rotting; also, frost-free models encourage drying-out. So the refrigerator is not an ideal place for storing garlic. However, it is good for storing peeled cloves or crushed or chopped garlic for up to a week if you put them in an airtight jar. Reduce tainting of uncovered food by keeping a small bowl of bicarbonate of soda (baking soda) in the refrigerator, stirring it every few days and replacing it every 2–3 months.

Inspect stored garlic frequently and remove any soft or mouldy bulbs or cloves. Separated cloves dry and rot faster, so break off only those you intend using immediately. Any crystals forming on stored garlic consist of the harmless garlic flavonoid allixin.

Preserving Garlic

While fresh garlic offers the best flavour and health benefits, preserved garlic is a useful standby and contains many health-promoting constituents. You can preserve garlic by drying, freezing, or steeping in oil, vinegar or wine.

Drying garlic

As garlic dries, its flavour intensifies. Garlic bulbs dry out in 4–10 months at room temperature. There are three methods of drying garlic faster:

- Dry 5mm/¼in thick slices at warm room temperature in a dry, well-ventilated, non-sunny space. They should dry out in 1–2 weeks.

- Use a food dehydrator according to its instructions.

- Dry cloves in the oven at no more than 50°C/122°F for several hours until dry and crisp. (Higher temperatures destroy alliinase.)

Keep dried garlic in an airtight container.

Freezing garlic

You can freeze garlic for several months as follows:

- Freeze peeled cloves in a plastic freezer bag. This changes the cloves' texture slightly.

- Freeze garlic juice in an ice-cube tray, then transfer the shapes into a plastic freezer bag.

- Freeze chopped garlic in a plastic freezer bag. When you want to use it, grate or break off what you need.

- Freeze peeled cloves covered with oil in a covered freezer container.

- Freeze crushed garlic mixed with extra-virgin olive oil (about 6 tbsp oil for the cloves from one medium bulb). Freeze this purée in a plastic freezer bag. When you want to use it, scrape off what you need.

Remember to label and date each batch.

Preserving garlic in oil

When garlic cloves or crushed garlic are immersed in oil, their oil-soluble flavour compounds gradually diffuse into the oil. This makes the garlic taste milder and imparts a garlicky scent to the oil, so it is good for incorporating into salad dressings or for cooking.

However, *Clostridium botulinum* bacterial spores from traces of soil on unpeeled cloves readily contaminate peeled cloves. Once whole or crushed cloves are immersed in oil, spores readily germinate because of the absence of air, the warmth of room temperature, the moisture in garlic and the lack of acidity. Germination produces botulinum toxin. Consuming botulinum can cause botulism within 10 days. Botulism can cause dizziness, blurred or double vision and, at worst, paralysis. In the US, botulism causes fewer than one in 400 cases of food poisoning, but it kills 8 in 100 affected people. Contamination with spores is much more likely in homemade garlic-in-oil than in commercially produced products (see below). You cannot detect botulinum by looking, smelling or tasting.

Germination of spores can be prevented with acidity, sugar, dryness and a low temperature (below 3°C/38°F). Regulations in the US and Canada require that garlic-in-oil offered for sale must be acidifed, contain salt or have other protection. In Australia, it must have a pH (acidity indicator) of below 4. Some commercial products are pressure-cooked to kill spores. Ordinary cooking does not work because heat kills spores only at 121°C/250°F for at least 3 minutes, which would spoil its flavour.

Buying preserved garlic in oil

If you buy garlic in oil, check that it contains acid or salt, refrigerate it when you get home and abide by the 'use-by' date.

Preserving garlic in oil at home

If you preserve garlic in oil, consume it immediately, or refrigerate it without delay and use within a week.

To preserve garlic cloves in oil at home so they can safely be stored, the US Food and Drug Administration recommends soaking them for 24 hours in vinegar, wine or a citric- or phosphoric-acid solution before draining them and covering them with oil. You can then keep them in the freezer for 6–10 months. However, the acid imparts a very particular flavour.

Another way of preserving garlic cloves in oil at home so they can safely be stored is to use cloves that have been thoroughly dehydrated (see page 39). Their moisture level is then less than 6 per cent and you can refrigerate them for a month. However, sulfur compounds don't diffuse out of dried garlic as well as from fresh garlic, so the oil doesn't have such a garlicky flavour.

Crushed garlic in oil

There are two ways of preparing this. One is to crush several cloves in a few tablespoons of extra-virgin olive oil to produce garlic oil-macerate. The oil keeps air from the alliinase released by crushing, so it cannot release allicin. Another way is to crush the cloves and leave them to stand for up to 90 minutes before adding oil. This produces increasingly more allicin within that timeframe. So the sooner you use it within 90 minutes, the milder the flavour, and vice versa.

Use crushed garlic in oil at once – for example, dribbled on pizzas 5 minutes before the end of the cooking time, or in a salad dressing. Alternatively, refrigerate and use within a week.

ROASTED GARLIC IN OIL

Roasted cloves have a mild sweet nutty flavour that gradually diffuses into oil.

6–8 whole garlic bulbs
600ml/21fl oz/scant 2½ cups extra-virgin olive oil
fresh thyme sprigs
2 bay leaves

Preheat the oven to 190°C/375°F/gas 5.

Put the unpeeled cloves on a sheet of aluminium foil on a baking tray, add a little oil and coat the cloves with it. Wrap the foil over the cloves to make a parcel. Roast for 30–40 minutes. Unwrap the foil and leave to cool.

Put the roasted cloves, thyme and bay leaves into a sterilized glass jar, cover with the remaining oil and refrigerate without delay.

When ready to use, remove however many cloves you need from the jar, snip the end off each one and squeeze out its soft flavourful inside. Use the oil for salad dressings or stir-fries, for example.

Use within a week.

Preserving garlic cloves in vinegar or wine

Peeled cloves preserved in plain or sweetened vinegar or wine taste good with cold meat or in stir-fries. The garlicky vinegar is good in salad dressings, soups and casseroles and the garlicky wine in soups and casseroles.

You get neither garlic breath nor secondary garlic odour from these cloves because they aren't damaged, so allicin and its derivatives are not produced. Instead, the garlic contains only odour-free water-soluble compounds. Gamma-glutamyl cysteine breaks down very slowly into S-allyl cysteine, which gradually diffuses into the vinegar. The amount of S-allyl cysteine therefore rises slowly in both the garlic and the vinegar.

Infiltration of the cloves by acid from the vinegar or wine inactivates their alliinase, so there is no allicin production even when the cloves are eventually chewed.

You can safely refrigerate garlic-in-vinegar or garlic-in-wine for about 4 months because vinegar and wine are acidic, which prevents germination of *Clostridium botulinum* spores (see page 35).

Garlic Products for Cooks

These include:

- Peeled raw garlic cloves – perhaps dressed with something acidic, or blanched.

- Garlic powder – ¼ teaspoon is equivalent to 1 medium-sized garlic clove. The flavour resembles that of boiled garlic. Garlic powder for cooking usually has a lower potential allicin yield than garlic powder in garlic-supplement tablets or capsules.

- Other dehydrated garlic – sliced as 'flakes', chopped as 'chips', or minced.

- Garlic paste – which may contain garlic powder, juice or oil mixed with vegetable oil, salt, dextrose, glycerine or acid.

- Crushed (minced) garlic – usually preserved with phosphoric acid.

- Frozen crushed garlic.

- Garlic cloves in oil.

- Garlic oil – which is steam-distilled garlic oil (see page 25) diluted with a cheaper vegetable oil.

- Garlic salt – this contains up to 81 per cent salt, 18–19 per cent garlic powder and 1–2 per cent calcium stearate (to prevent clumping). 1 tablespoon equates to 1 medium garlic clove. To make garlic salt, whizz dried garlic in a blender until powdered. Add 4 parts salt to 1 part garlic powder and blend for 2 seconds. Use garlic salt sparingly, bearing in mind health advice to limit daily salt intake.

- Pickled garlic – a popular presentation in China and Russia, for example.

- Fermented garlic cloves – which are black because fermentation produces the black pigment melanoidin.

Such products are convenient, but depending on what's been done to them, many contain no alliinase or are lower in allicin or allicin-derivatives than the equivalent amount of fresh garlic (see also page 10).

Garlic Remedies

Some people make their own garlic remedies for the sake of cost and availability, or because they want to use home-grown garlic. Options include garlic syrup, garlic water, garlic-powder capsules and garlic tea.

Garlic syrup
This may ease a cough or sore throat (see page 100).

> 100g/3½oz/heaped ⅓ cup caster (superfine) sugar
> 100g/3½oz garlic cloves, peeled
> optional: few drops of orange, lemon or cinnamon oil

Put 100ml/3½fl oz/scant ½ cup water into a pan, add the sugar and garlic and heat gently until the sugar dissolves. Bring the syrup to the boil, then remove from the heat. Leave to cool, then strain. Flavour with orange, lemon or cinnamon oil, if you like.

Garlic water

This is less likely than crushed garlic to irritate the skin.

Make it by mixing one part of garlic juice (see page 31) with 3 to 4 parts of water. Alternatively, stir a crushed clove into half a glass of water, wait 30–60 minutes for some allicin to develop, then use the garlicky water.

To treat a large area of skin (for example, for widespread psoriasis), leave 6 crushed cloves to stand for 30–60 minutes then add to your bath water – perhaps with some peppermint leaves to freshen the smell. Soak in it for half an hour.

Garlic-powder capsules

Buy empty animal- or vegetable-gelatine capsules from a health-food store or on the internet. Dry the cloves from several garlic bulbs (see page 8) then crush them using a pestle and mortar or in a spice mill. Fill the capsules with the garlic powder. Keep in an airtight container.

Garlic tea

For alliin-rich tea, add one peeled garlic clove to a cup of just-boiled water and let it steep for 5 minutes. Sweeten with honey or sugar if desired.

For tea rich in allicin and allicin derivatives, let a crushed garlic clove stand for 60–90 minutes. Add it to a cup of just-boiled water and let it steep for 5 minutes. Sweeten with honey or sugar if desired.

Garlic Breath

Suggestions for reducing garlic breath include:

- Adding milk to garlic before cooking it (recent research found this halved the expected intensity of garlic breath).

- Drinking 200ml/7fl oz/generous ¾ cup milk before or during a garlic-containing meal.

- Chewing raw fruits or vegetables, herbs such as mint or basil (parsley doesn't help), or caraway, fennel or cardamom seeds.

- Eating cooked rice or eggs.

- Cleaning teeth to remove garlic debris.

- Mouth-washing with half a glass of water containing a teaspoon of bicarbonate of soda.

- Using a commercial mouthwash.

You can reduce your sensitivity to another person's garlic breath by eating garlic when they do.

Blue or Turquoise Discoloration

A blue or turquoise colour sometimes develops in chopped or crushed garlic, which, although safe, can be offputting. The three possible explanations are outlined below.

One is that the cysteine sulfoxide iso-alliin breaks down into thiosulfinates, which react with a garlic amino acid to produce up to eight blue and green pigments. Cloves with high levels of this amino acid are more likely to change colour. The coloration is most intense in an acidic environment (such as with lemon juice, vinegar or tomato). It's also encouraged by refrigerating garlic or by pickling slightly unripe garlic. In northern China, cloves from long-stored garlic are immersed in vinegar for a week to make them into vivid green 'Laba' pickled garlic, which is eaten with dumplings at Chinese New Year.

Another possibility is that an enzyme in raw garlic reacts with garlic's sulfur, and with traces of copper in water, or in aluminium, cast-iron or tin utensils, or in vinegar or lemon juice, to create blue copper sulphate.

A third explanation is that the iodine in iodized table salt 'blues' garlic; this can be avoided by using canning or kosher salt.

Irradiated Garlic

More than 50 countries allow garlic to be treated with ionising radiation (gamma, X-ray or electron radiation) to destroy insects, kill bacteria and fungi (to prevent rotting) and prevent sprouting (to increase shelf-life). Irradiation does not kill viruses or destroy bacterial toxins.

Irradiated garlic must be labelled as such in many countries, including the US and European-Union countries.

If you are not sure whether a bulb has been irradiated, you can get a good idea by cutting a clove in half. If it has not been irradiated, the growing area down the centre will be creamy or greenish-white. If it has been irradiated, then depending on how long ago this was done, this area may already have turned brown.

It is sometimes suggested that irradiation inactivates alliinase and other enzymes in garlic, but this is not true.

CHAPTER 4

Recipes

The irreplaceable flavour of garlic varies according to the variety and growing conditions of the plant (see page 1) and how the garlic is prepared (see page 10).

When using garlic, be guided by the tips in Chapter 3. Cooked and raw garlic have different flavour and health-benefit profiles. Asians mostly eat garlic cooked, whereas Americans, Australians and Europeans often eat it raw, as well as cooked. Whether you use garlic raw or cooked, note the following points:

- Whole cloves, raw or cooked, contain no allicin or allicin derivatives, so their flavour is milder (meaning less 'hot' or pungent) and less rich than that of crushed or chopped garlic.

- Crushing or chopping garlic initiates allicin production, which peaks 90 minutes later. So the longer (up to 90 minutes) you leave crushed or chopped cloves before use, the more pungent and 'garlicky' their flavour.

- Certain varieties of garlic (such as Silverskins and Porcelains) contain relatively more allicin, so their flavour is potentially hotter.

- To gain the benefits from the flavours of both cooked and raw garlic, add crushed or chopped garlic at or near the beginning of cooking, then again towards or at the end.

Raw garlic tips: note that adding vinegar or lemon juice to chopped or crushed cloves stops allicin production. Waiting for more or less time within 90 minutes of crushing or chopping encourages more or less pungency, depending on how much allicin has been produced.

Crushed raw garlic is excellent in salad dressings, or sprinkled on pizzas just before the end of their cooking time, or tossed with a little extra-virgin olive oil into freshly cooked and drained spinach or other vegetables.

If you prefer just a hint of raw garlic, rub the cut surface of a clove around a salad bowl before adding the salad leaves, or around a fondue pan before adding the cheese.

Cooked garlic tips: note that cooking crushed or chopped cloves stops allicin production. Waiting for more or less time within 90 minutes after crushing or chopping encourages more or less pungency, depending on how much allicin has been produced.

Cooking crushed or chopped cloves speeds allicin's breakdown, making garlic's flavour more complex and less pungent.

Roasting whole unpeeled cloves (page 37) adds sweetish nutty caramel flavours.

Young garlic bulbs

'Young wet' garlic bulbs are newly matured but not dried. They have a fresh mild flavour and a soft texture.

Spring garlic and green garlic

Spring garlic tastes mildly garlicky and you can eat it all. It's good chopped and added raw to salads or stir-fried with other vegetables.

Green garlic (see page 4) has a mild fresh flavour and is excellent steamed or added to stir-fries and casseroles.

Stalks and flowers

Garlic stalks can be boiled for 5 minutes, or chopped and either stir-fried or added to a casserole. You can eat garlic flowers raw (for example, in salads, or dressed with olive oil and lemon juice) or cooked (for example, in an omelette).

In the following recipes, please note:

- Each recipe serves 4.

- 1 tsp (teaspoon) = 5ml; 1 tbsp (tablespoon) = 15ml; 1 cup = 240ml/8fl oz

- Garlic cloves vary in size by tenfold or more; a medium-sized clove weighs 4g/just over $^1/_{10}$ oz.

- Eggs are medium (US large) unless otherwise stated.

- If using a fan oven, reduce the temperature in the recipe by 20°C/35°F.

- Salt is included only when needed to cure or soften other ingredients. Anyone who wants salt for flavour can add it at the table.

- If you like only a little garlic, add fewer cloves than the recipe specifies.

Starters (Appetizers)

Garlic adds moreishness to hot Anchovy dip (see page 50), is vital for the colourful cold soup Gazpacho (see page 51) and is traditional in recipes such as Basturma (see page 48) and Bruschetta (see page 48). You can also lightly grill (broil) slices of baguette spread with butter containing crushed raw garlic or, if you prefer a milder flavour, crushed boiled cloves or the squeezed-out centres of cloves roasted in their skins.

GARLICKY OIL FOR DIPPING

Dipping good crusty bread into garlic-flavoured oil makes a great starter.

> 120ml/4fl oz/½ cup extra-virgin olive oil
> 2–3 garlic cloves, thinly sliced
> ground black pepper
> grated rind of ½ lemon (optional)
> bread, for dipping

Put the olive oil and garlic into a small pan and heat gently until the garlic begins to sizzle. Remove from the heat and leave to stand for 20 minutes. Remove the garlic slices. Stir in black pepper to taste, plus the lemon rind, if using. Pour the garlicky oil into a bowl and serve with the bread.

Store any leftover oil in the refrigerator for up to 1 week.

BRUSCHETTA

The better the bread, olive oil and tomatoes, the more delectable the bruschetta. Thin slices of air-dried ham (such as Parma ham and other prosciutto from Italy; Bayonne ham from the Basque-country area of France; and Serrano ham and other *jamón* from Spain) are a good alternative to tomatoes as a topping.

    4 thick slices of good crusty bread
    4 garlic cloves, peeled
    4 tbsp extra-virgin olive oil
    4 large firm ripe tomatoes, sliced
    ground black pepper
    small handful of basil, roughly chopped (optional)

Toast the bread. Rub each garlic clove very firmly over one side of each slice of toast, so the clove disintegrates (but do not rub so firmly that the bread disintegrates). Pour 1 tbsp of olive oil evenly over each slice of bread, then top with the tomatoes. Season with black pepper to taste, and sprinkle with basil, if using.

BASTURMA

This cured meat originated in Turkey and is prized for its flavour. Beef (or lamb) is salted, washed, dried and spiced, then dried again. Basturma's Italian cousin, pastrami, has different flavourings. Serve basturma simply thinly sliced; alternatively, grill (broil) it or fry it in olive oil. It's also excellent in sandwiches or on pizzas, makes a delicious lunch when added to an omelette accompanied by pitta bread, and can also have beans added to it to make a main course.

900g/2lb beef fillet, in one piece

175g/6oz/½ cup salt

8 garlic cloves, peeled

3 tbsp ground fenugreek

3 tbsp paprika

2 tsp cayenne pepper

2 tsp ground cumin

2 tsp ground black pepper

Put the beef into a large roasting tin and sprinkle with the salt. Cover with clingfilm (plastic wrap). Place heavy weights (such as cans of food) on top. Put the beef into a cool, dry, dark place (such as a frost-free refrigerator) to cure for 4 days. Each day pour off the liquid that has accumulated and replenish the covering of salt when necessary. After 2 days, turn the beef over and re-salt.

Remove the beef, wash in cold running water, and dry with a cloth.

Put the beef on a metal rack in the roasting tin. Leave to dry in a cool, dry, dark place for 7 days.

Crush the garlic and put it into a bowl with the fenugreek, paprika, cayenne pepper, cumin and black pepper, then add 210ml/7fl oz/generous ¾ cup cold water and stir to make a paste. Smooth the paste all over the beef. Now put the beef on a clean rack in the roasting tin and leave in the cool, dry, dark place for 2 weeks.

Finally, wipe off the remaining paste.

ANCHOVY DIP

Crisp fresh raw vegetables (crudités) are turned into a sumptuous treat when accompanied by this famous Italian dip, also called *bagna cauda*.

4 tbsp extra-virgin olive oil
50g/2oz/½ stick butter
5 garlic cloves, peeled
85g/3oz canned anchovy fillets in oil
6 tbsp double (heavy) cream
ground black pepper

Serve with: fresh raw vegetables, such as celery, bell peppers, crisp lettuce, courgettes (zucchini), cauliflower and chicory (endive), cut into pieces.

Heat the oil and butter in a small pan. Add the garlic and anchovies and fry gently for about 4 minutes or until soft. Put the mixture into a blender, add the cream and black pepper and whizz until smooth.

Serve hot in a warmed bowl or a chafing dish (a bowl or pan over a flame or other heat source), and offer the vegetables and, perhaps, good crusty bread, separately.

GAZPACHO

This chilled red soup, with its colourful garnish and crunchy croutons, is just right on a summer's day.

For the soup
450g/1lb tomatoes, chopped
425g/15oz tinned (canned) plum tomatoes in tomato juice
1 small green bell pepper, deseeded and chopped
3 tbsp apple cider or balsamic vinegar
4 tbsp extra-virgin olive oil
small cucumber, peeled and chopped
1 small onion, peeled and chopped
2 garlic cloves, peeled and crushed
1 tsp paprika
1 slice white bread, crusts removed

To garnish
garlic croutons (see page 80)
½ small cucumber, peeled, deseeded and chopped
small yellow or orange bell pepper, deseeded and chopped

Put all the soup ingredients and 180ml/6fl oz/¾ cup water into a blender and whizz until smooth. Refrigerate the soup for several hours, then serve with the garnishes.

CHICKEN AND GARLIC SOUP

This soup restores flagging spirits and health. Cooking garlic cloves unpeeled enriches the stock with quercetin. Italian cooks refer to the celery, carrots, onions and garlic in this recipe as *odori* because of their fragrance.

For the stock
1.3kg/3lb chicken pieces
1 carrot
2 celery stalks
1 onion
12 garlic cloves, unpeeled
6 bay leaves

For the soup
pan of stock, cooked vegetables and chicken, from the recipe
    above
4 carrots, chopped
3 celery stalks, chopped
2 onions, chopped
6 garlic cloves, peeled and chopped
salt and ground black pepper
120ml/4fl oz/½ cup single (light) cream (optional)

Put all stock ingredients into a large pan with 1.45 litres/48fl oz/6 cups water. Bring to the boil and simmer for 1 hour.

Remove the chicken pieces with a slotted spoon and put them on to a plate to cool. Strip the meat from the bones and put it on a plate.

Remove the garlic, snip off one end of each clove and squeeze its contents into the pan. Remove the vegetables with a slotted spoon and put them in a blender, but don't whizz them yet.

Let the pan of stock cool, then skim off the fat. (You can put this into a bowl and keep it in the refrigerator for some other recipe.)

To make the soup, add the carrots, celery, onions and garlic to the pan of stock. Bring to the boil and simmer for 15 minutes.

Put a cupful of this soup into the blender that contains the cooked vegetables from the stock recipe, and whizz. Add this blended mixture, plus the remaining stock and the cooked chicken, to the pan of soup and season with salt and black pepper to taste.

Bring the soup to the boil, stirring, and simmer, covered, for 15 minutes. Add cream, if using.

Vegetables and Salads

Garlic complements most vegetables. Here you'll find two recipes for vegetables cooked with garlic and two for salads scented with garlic.

GARLICKY MASHED POTATOES

Boiling the potatoes is quick and easy, but if you have the time to bake them, you will get a particularly good flavour. Adding fried or roasted garlic gives a mild nutty garlicky flavour. Finally, adding white sauce and cream makes the garlicky mash sumptuously smooth. If you're short of time, omit the white sauce and add a little extra cream instead.

675g/1½lb potatoes

For the fried or roasted garlic
20 garlic cloves, unpeeled
25g/1oz/½ stick butter (for frying) or 2 tbsp extra-virgin olive
    oil (for roasting)

For the white sauce
40g/1½oz/3 tbsp butter
2 tbsp plain (all-purpose) flour
180ml/6fl oz/¾ cup milk, warmed

120ml/4fl oz/½ cup single (light) cream
pinch of ground black pepper
handful of fresh parsley, finely chopped

For boiled potatoes, peel the potatoes and boil in a pan of water for 15–20 minutes, or until tender, then drain and put into a bowl. Meanwhile, put the garlic into a small pan with the butter and fry gently for 10 minutes, or until tender, taking care not to let the garlic brown. When cool enough to handle, snip the tips off with scissors and squeeze the soft centres into the bowl of potatoes.

For baked potatoes, preheat the oven to 180°C/350°F/gas 4 and bake the potatoes in their skins for 1½ hours. Remove them from the oven and scrape their insides into a bowl. 30 minutes before the potatoes are ready, roast the garlic in the olive oil (see page 37), then squeeze the soft garlic into the bowl.

Make the white sauce by melting the butter in a small saucepan, then adding the flour and stirring over a low heat for 2 minutes. Add the milk gradually and continue stirring until the sauce is thick and smooth.

Either mash the potatoes and cooked garlic or, for a smoother texture, put them through a potato ricer. Stir in the white sauce and cream, season with pepper and sprinkle with parsley.

SPINACH WITH CREAM AND GARLIC

Boiling the garlic makes it taste mild and gives it a soft crunchiness similar to that of flaked almonds.

900g/2lb/18 cups firmly packed spinach
8 garlic cloves, peeled
150ml/5fl oz/generous ½ cup double (heavy) cream

Wash the spinach leaves well and put them into the top of a steamer with water in its pan. Put the lid on and steam gently for 1–2 minutes or until the spinach has collapsed and is soft enough to eat.

Put the garlic and 150ml/5fl oz/generous ½ cup water into a small pan and simmer for 5–10 minutes, or until softened. Drain and leave until cool enough to handle, then slice the cloves thinly along their length.

Empty the water from the steamer pan and put the spinach into it. Stir in the sliced garlic and the cream, then heat through thoroughly before serving.

BROAD BEAN AND GARLIC SALAD

Fresh or frozen broad (fava) beans are ideal for this salad, but tinned (canned) ones are good too.

> 225g/8oz shelled broad (fava) beans, defrosted if frozen,
>   drained if tinned (canned)
> 2 garlic cloves, peeled and crushed
> 150ml/5fl oz/generous ½ cup plain bio-yoghurt
> 2 tsp lemon juice
> small handful of fresh parsley, chopped
> small handful of fresh dill, chopped

Cook the fresh or frozen broad beans in boiling water until tender, then drain. Put into a large bowl and leave to cool. (If using tinned beans, just tip into a bowl.)

Put the garlic, yoghurt and lemon juice into a small bowl and stir, then pour the dressing over the beans and stir.

Add most of the parsley and dill and stir again. Sprinkle the remainder on top. Serve with garlic bread as a starter or with cold meat as a main course.

CAESAR SALAD

This makes a first-class starter as it is, or can be turned into an excellent main course by adding 75–100g/3–4oz of cold cooked chicken.

1 garlic clove, unpeeled and halved lengthways
1 large crispy lettuce such as Cos (Romaine), Webb or Iceberg, washed, trimmed, torn into pieces and patted dry with kitchen paper
ground black pepper
3 tbsp olive oil
2 eggs
2 tsp fresh lemon juice
8 tinned (canned) anchovy fillets in oil, drained and each cut into four pieces
50g/2oz Parmesan cheese, shaved or coarsely grated
garlic croutons made with 4 slices of bread (see page 80)

Rub the cut surfaces of the garlic clove around the inside of a large salad bowl. Add the lettuce, black pepper to taste, and olive oil and toss gently until the lettuce is well coated with oil.

Put the eggs into a pan of water and bring it to the boil, then cook for 3 minutes. Remove the eggs and leave to cool a little, then remove the shell and cut into quarters lengthwise. Arrange the egg quarters on top of the salad, sprinkle with the lemon juice and anchovies and toss gently. Add the Parmesan and croutons before serving.

Sauces, Toppings and Dressings

These garlic-flavoured sauces, toppings and dressings are based on traditional recipes and can transform many main courses, salads and vegetable dishes into something special.

GARLIC MAYONNAISE

This sauce originated in Provence and is also called aïoli ('garlic and oil'). This recipe is quick, easy and reliable. It's an excellent dip for raw peppers, radishes, courgettes (zucchini), celery, cucumber, tomatoes and other crudités. It's also good with cold cooked prawns (shrimp) or hard-boiled eggs; in hamburgers; and with baked potatoes.

Four variations are almond skordalia (good with cold cooked asparagus, French beans, carrots or beetroot); green herb and garlic mayonnaise; rouille (traditionally added to fish soup); and remoulade.

1 large (US extra large) egg
6 garlic cloves
1 tsp Dijon mustard
pinch of caster (superfine) sugar
pinch of ground black pepper
300ml/10½fl oz/1¼ cups extra-virgin olive oil
2 tbsp fresh lemon juice

Put the egg, garlic, mustard, sugar, black pepper and 4 tbsp of the oil into a blender and whizz until smooth. Continue to whizz while slowly adding 150ml/5fl oz/generous ½ cup of the oil and all the lemon juice, followed by the remaining oil. Add 1 tbsp boiling water and whizz briefly; repeat if you prefer your mayonnaise to be less thick.

If covered with clingfilm (plastic wrap), this mayonnaise and its variations will keep in the refrigerator for 2–3 days.

For almond skordalia: add 1 tbsp fresh white breadcrumbs, 1 tbsp ground almonds, 1 tbsp finely chopped parsley and a pinch of cayenne pepper. Whizz briefly.

For green herb and garlic mayonnaise: add a handful of finely chopped mixed herbs (such as parsley, tarragon, chervil or lovage), and a small handful of fresh spinach, boiled in water for a few minutes until tender, then sieved. Whizz briefly.

For rouille: add 1 tsp cayenne pepper and 2 tbsp plus 2 tsp tomato purée. Whizz briefly.

For remoulade: add 2 tsp horseradish sauce, 1 tsp yellow mustard, 1 tsp hot sauce (such as Tabasco), 1 tsp Worcestershire sauce, 2 tbsp chopped spring onion (scallion) tops, 2 tbsp chopped parsley and 2 tbsp capers. Whizz briefly.

WALNUT AND GARLIC SAUCE

This sauce originated in Toulouse in France and is excellent with raw or cooked vegetables, pasta, or cold fish or meat.

Walnuts are rich in the healthy fats that can help to reduce the levels of 'bad' cholesterol in the blood, and also contain manganese and B vitamins.

3 garlic cloves
225g/8oz/2¼ cups shelled walnuts
4 tbsp walnut oil
120ml/4fl oz/½ cup double (heavy) cream
2 tbsp finely chopped parsley

Put the garlic and walnuts into a blender and whizz until well blended. Gradually pour in the oil and then the cream, with the blender at medium speed. Put the sauce into a bowl and stir in the parsley.

PARSLEY AND GARLIC DRESSING

This is particularly popular in France, Greece, Québec and the southern states of the US. Its French name, *persillade*, comes from *persil*, for parsley. Adding lemon zest makes it into a lemony dressing called gremolata; a further addition of fresh breadcrumbs means it can be used for a crust topping.

The flavours of *persillade* and gremolata marry superbly with grilled (broiled) or barbecued fish or meat.

Another option is to add fresh breadcrumbs then to use the mixture as a coating for meat, for example, 15 minutes before the end of cooking, to create a 'crust'.

4–8 garlic cloves, peeled and crushed
2 handfuls of flat-leaf parsley, lightly chopped
zest and juice of 1 lemon (optional, for gremolata)
2 tbsp fresh breadcrumbs (optional, for crust topping)

Lightly mix the garlic and parsley together in a bowl and sprinkle over grilled (broiled), fried or barbecued meat, chicken or fish, or even boiled or roast potatoes.

For gremolata, add the lemon zest and juice and mix to combine.
For a crust topping, incorporate the breadcrumbs and sprinkle the mixture over the top of grilled or oven-baked meat, chicken or fish 15 minutes before the end of cooking time. Serve within an hour.

GARLIC AND ANCHOVY SAUCE

This sauce thickens best if its ingredients start at room temperature.
It's easiest to use a blender, though traditionally it is made using a
pestle and mortar and served from the mortar. Use it on watercress
or chicory salads or on pasta, or serve it with crusty rustic bread.

2–3 garlic cloves, peeled
120ml/4fl oz/½ cup olive oil
8 tinned (canned) anchovy fillets in oil, drained
1 tsp lemon juice

Either put the ingredients into a blender and whizz until smooth,
or put the garlic into a mortar, crush with a pestle, then slowly pour
in the oil, stirring constantly. Add the anchovies and lemon juice,
mash with a fork, then grind with the pestle.

Pasta and Pizza

Garlic is a vital ingredient of many pasta sauces and pizza toppings.

PASTA WITH GARLIC AND OIL

Italians call pasta dressed with garlic and olive oil *aglio e olio* or just *aio e oio*. It's a favourite even for sophisticated palates. Cook the pasta *al dente* so it retains some firmness.

   450g/1lb dried or 600g/1lb 4oz fresh pasta
   120ml/4fl oz/½ cup extra-virgin olive oil
   2 garlic cloves, peeled and crushed
   ground black pepper
   small handful of chopped parsley or oregano (optional)
   50g/2oz Parmesan or pecorino cheese, grated (optional)

Cook the dried pasta as directed on the packet, or fresh pasta for 2–3 minutes until it floats to the surface. Drain well and return to the pan. Stir in the olive oil, garlic and black pepper to taste.

Stir in the parsley or oregano, and grated cheese, if using.

PIZZA WITH GARLIC AND BASIL

Using half wholemeal (wholewheat) bread flour and half white bread flour produces a slightly nutty-flavoured pizza. Possible additions to the topping include anchovy fillets, pitted black olives, marinated artichoke hearts and crispy bacon.

225g/8oz/1½ cups wholemeal (wholewheat) bread flour
225g/8oz/heaped 1¾ cups white bread flour
7g/¼oz sachet (envelope) dried yeast
1 tsp salt
1 tbsp clear honey or caster (superfine) sugar
6 tbsp extra-virgin olive oil
2 onions, peeled and chopped
350g/12oz tomatoes, chopped
10 garlic cloves, peeled and crushed
2 tsp dried mixed herbs
pinch of ground black pepper
300g/11oz mozzarella cheese, thinly sliced
small handful of basil leaves

Put the flours, yeast, salt and honey or sugar into a large mixing bowl and make a well in the centre. Pour 1 tbsp of the olive oil and 300ml/10fl oz/1¼ cups lukewarm water into the well and mix into the dry ingredients. Add a little more lukewarm water if necessary to make the dough bind together easily into a kneadable ball. Knead by hand or using the dough hook of a food mixer for 10 minutes. Cover with a damp cloth and leave to rise in a warm, draft-free place for 2 hours or until doubled in size.

Pour 3 tbsp of the oil into a frying pan, add the onions and fry gently, stirring occasionally, for about 10 minutes. Add the tomatoes, garlic, dried herbs and pepper and fry gently for 15–20 minutes, stirring as often as necessary to prevent the tomatoes sticking to the pan.

Roll the dough into a circle about 5mm/¼in thick. If you prefer, you can divide the dough into two pieces and roll each into a circle about 5mm/¼in thick. Transfer to a baking tray and prick all over with a fork. Leave to rise a little for 30 minutes in a warm place.

Preheat the oven to 240°C/475°F/gas 9, then turn the oven down to 200°C/400°F/gas 6 and put the pizza in. Bake for about 15 minutes, or until you see that the crust is golden-brown and crispy underneath when you lift up part of its edge.

Remove from the oven, lay the mozzarella slices on top and sprinkle with the remaining oil. Return the pizza to the oven and bake for 10 minutes to melt the mozzarella. Remove, sprinkle with the basil and serve at once.

PASTA SALAD WITH GARLIC SAUSAGE AND SUNDRIED TOMATOES

Different pasta shapes taste different, probably because some retain more dressing than others and each has a particular mouth-feel.

Ring the changes by adding toasted pine nuts, finely sliced yellow (bell) pepper or coarsely grated raw courgettes (zucchini).

225g/8oz/2 cups dried pasta shapes

2 tsp extra-virgin olive oil

100g/3½oz sundried tomatoes, thinly sliced

175g/6oz garlic sausage, thinly sliced then cut into strips

2 garlic cloves, peeled and crushed

150ml/5fl oz/⅔ cup mayonnaise

1 tbsp single (light) cream

175g/6oz/1¼ cups button mushrooms, sliced

ground black pepper

2 spring onions (scallions), chopped

Put the pasta, olive oil and half the sundried tomatoes into a pan of water and boil according to the directions on the packet until the pasta is al dente. Drain and put into a large bowl to cool.

Meanwhile, put the garlic sausage into a non-stick pan and fry for 10 minutes or until crisp. Drain on kitchen paper and cool.

Stir the garlic sausage, garlic, mayonnaise, cream, mushrooms, the boiled sun-dried tomato, the other sundried tomatoes and black pepper to taste, into the cold cooked pasta. Sprinkle with the spring onions.

Eggs, Meat and Poultry

Among these recipes are some unusual ones, such as Eggs with green garlic shoots (see page 68), Seared garlic beef (see page 69) and Lamb's hearts with lemon, garlic and parsley (see page 71).

TUNISIAN LAMB

This typical Tunisian dish is flavoured with garlic and spices and sweetened with dried fruits.

    4 tbsp extra-virgin olive oil
    2 onions, sliced
    2 carrots, sliced
    900g/2lb boneless leg or shoulder of lamb, cubed
    4 garlic cloves, peeled and crushed
    1 small red chilli pepper, deseeded and very finely chopped
    1 tsp ground coriander
    ½ tsp caraway seeds, ground
    1 red bell pepper, sliced
    100g/3½oz/heaped ½ cup shelled broad (fava) beans
    50g/2oz/heaped ¼ cup dried pitted apricots
    50g/2oz/scant ¼ cup dried pitted prunes
    50g/2oz/scant ½ cup sultanas (golden raisins)
    850g/1lb 14oz tinned (canned) chickpeas (garbanzo beans)

Heat 2 tbsp of the olive oil in a large casserole on the hob then add the onions and carrots and fry, stirring frequently, until just coloured. Put the onions and carrots into a bowl.

Now heat the remaining olive oil in the casserole and add the lamb, garlic, chilli, coriander and ground caraway seeds. Fry for 5–7 minutes, stirring frequently, until the lamb starts to brown.

Add 570ml/20fl oz/generous 2¼ cups water, the red pepper and broad beans, bring to the boil and simmer for 40 minutes, adding more water if necessary to keep the lamb just covered in liquid. Add the apricots, prunes and sultanas, then bring back to the boil and simmer for 30 minutes. Add the chickpeas and heat through for 2–3 minutes.

Serve with couscous to soak up the juices.

EGGS WITH GREEN GARLIC SHOOTS

Green garlic shoots impart a delicate flavour and are particularly good when cooked with eggs. This recipe is for butter-fried eggs, but a garlic-shoot omelette is just as fine.

115g/4oz/1 stick butter
12 garlic shoots, finely chopped
8 eggs

Put the butter into a large frying pan and heat until just sizzling. Add the garlic shoots and cook for 1 minute, stirring. Carefully break the eggs into the pan and cook until their whites are set, basting them with butter several times.

Serve with wholegrain bread.

SEARED GARLIC BEEF

This Korean recipe calls for a tender cut such as fillet or well-marbled sirloin. Slice it thinly with a very sharp knife or ask the butcher to do this for you. Cook the meat for no longer than 20 seconds per side or it will be overdone.

4 tbsp soy sauce

2 tbsp caster (superfine) sugar

12 garlic cloves, peeled and crushed

2 tbsp sesame oil, plus a little more for cooking the steak

8 thin slices of fillet or well-marbled beef sirloin, each about
75g/3oz

Put the soy sauce, sugar, garlic and sesame oil into a large bowl and stir to make the marinade.

Add the slices of steak and coat them with the marinade. Set aside for 3–4 hours. Remove the steak and wipe off the marinade with kitchen paper.

Brush the base of a large pan (ideally a ridged, heavy-based, cast-iron one) with sesame oil and then add the slices of steak and sear them for 10-20 seconds on each side, depending on whether you want them rare or medium rare. Alternatively, sear the steak on a barbecue for 10–20 seconds per side.

Serve with rice and fried aubergines (eggplant) or other vegetables.

STIR-FRIED PORK, PRAWNS AND CABBAGE

Inspired by recipes from Thailand, this is quick and easy to cook and goes well with rice.

3 tbsp toasted sesame oil

8 garlic cloves, peeled and crushed

225g/8oz lean pork, cut into 1cm/½in cubes

225g/8oz small prawns (shrimp)

325g/12oz green cabbage leaves, finely sliced and with the main vein removed

1 tsp caster (superfine) sugar

1 tbsp soy sauce

pinch of ground black pepper

Heat the oil in a wok or a deep-sided frying pan. Add the garlic and fry, stirring with a wooden spoon, for 1–2 minutes, until just beginning to brown. Add the pork and fry, stirring, for 5–6 minutes or until cooked through. Turn up the heat, add the prawns, cabbage, sugar, soy sauce and black pepper and cook, stirring, for 4–5 minutes.

LAMB'S HEARTS WITH LEMON, GARLIC AND PARSLEY

Well-trimmed heart meat is lean, flavourful and well partnered by garlic, parsley and, perhaps, lemon.

4 lamb's hearts, their fat and blood vessels trimmed off

6 tbsp extra-virgin olive oil

8 garlic cloves, peeled and crushed

2 slices of wholemeal (wholewheat) bread, made into
  breadcrumbs

large handful of flat-leaved parsley

1 lemon, quartered and trimmed, to garnish

Slice the hearts finely with a very sharp knife. Pour the olive oil into a large frying pan (ideally a heavy-based one) and heat gently. Add the sliced hearts and fry for 7–10 minutes or until well browned (but not burnt). Add the garlic and fry for 3 minutes more. Now stir in the breadcrumbs and parsley.

Serve hot, garnished with the lemon quarters.

CHICKEN WITH 40 CLOVES OF GARLIC

Forty is the traditional number of cloves for this French recipe, but some cooks fill the entire cavity of a chicken with garlic bulbs.

    2 or more bulbs of garlic, separated into cloves
    75g/3oz/¾ stick butter
    1.3kg/3lb chicken at room temperature
    2 tbsp extra-virgin olive oil
    ground black pepper
    1 tsp dried (or 1 tbsp fresh) thyme or tarragon

Preheat the oven to 180°C/350°F/gas 4.

Snip the ends from the garlic cloves with scissors, then put the cloves and 2 tablespoons of the butter into the cavity of the chicken. Put the remaining butter into a roasting tin. Put the chicken breast-side-down into the tin. Coat the chicken with the olive oil and sprinkle with a pinch of pepper.

Roast the chicken for 1 hour, basting every 20 minutes. Then turn it breast-side-up and roast for a further 30 minutes. Baste it, sprinkle with thyme or tarragon, and roast for a further 10 minutes, or until the skin is browned. Test that the chicken is cooked by inserting a skewer into a leg and checking that the juices run clear, not pink.

Either serve the garlic cloves with the chicken so each diner can squeeze out the sweet nutty insides, or squeeze their insides into the pan juices, stir, and serve separately.

Fish and Shellfish

The flavour of garlic goes well with that of most fish and shellfish.

SEA BASS WITH LEMON, GARLIC AND CORIANDER

The Moroccan marinade chermoula gives this dish a wonderful zing.
Red snapper, cod and haddock are good alternatives to sea bass.

large handful of coriander (cilantro) leaves
handful of parsley
3 garlic cloves, peeled
juice of 1 lemon
3 tbsp extra-virgin olive oil
½ tsp ground cumin
pinch of ground coriander
½ tsp paprika

4 sea-bass fillets, each weighing 175–225g/6–8oz

Put all the ingredients except for the fish into a blender and whizz
until smooth.

Put the fish into a large shallow baking dish and coat with the
marinade. Cover and put in the refrigerator for several hours or
overnight.

Preheat the grill (broiler) and place the oven-rack so the fish
will be about 10cm/4in below the grill. Grill (broil) the fish for 4–5
minutes.

MEDITERRANEAN FISH SOUP

This rich soup, also called bouillabaisse, is particularly good when accompanied by rouille (see page 59), grated Gruyère cheese and fried French bread.

4 tbsp extra-virgin olive oil

1 large red onion, peeled and chopped

2 carrots, peeled and chopped

2 celery sticks, finely chopped

4 garlic cloves, peeled and crushed

550g/1¼lb fish fillets, skinned, cleaned and cut into large chunks

2 tbsp tomato purée (paste)

300ml/10½fl oz/1¼ cups white wine

small handful of fresh mixed herbs

fish stock cube

pinch of ground black pepper

pinch of cayenne pepper

a few threads of saffron

To serve

½ recipe quantity rouille (see page 59)

100g/3½oz Gruyère cheese, finely grated

8 thin slices of French bread, fried until golden in 4 tbsp extra-virgin olive oil

Heat the oil in a large pan, add the onion, carrots and celery and fry for 5 minutes or until just beginning to brown. Add the garlic and cook gently for a further 2 minutes. Add the fish, tomato purée, wine, herbs, fish stock cube, pepper, cayenne pepper and 900ml/30fl oz/3½ cups water and simmer, with the mixture bubbling gently, for 35 minutes.

Either put the mixture through a sieve or liquidize it in a blender. Return it to the pan and heat gently until bubbling. Stir in the saffron and serve, offering the rouille, Gruyère cheese and fried bread separately.

MUSSELS WITH GARLIC AND CREAM

Mussels cooked with cream, parsley and garlic are a taste of heaven. Using an empty mussel shell to pincer mussels from other shells is the traditional way to eat mussels, but you'll need a bowl of warm water containing lemon juice to rinse your fingers afterwards.

1.8kg/4lb mussels in their shells
4 tbsp extra-virgin olive oil
1 onion, finely chopped
2 garlic cloves, peeled and crushed
3 bay leaves
150ml/5fl oz/scant ⅔ cup dry white wine
pinch of nutmeg
120ml/4fl oz/½ cup double (heavy) cream
small handful of fresh parsley, chopped
country bread, to serve

Debeard and clean the mussels. Discard any that do not shut when tapped.

Heat the olive oil in a pan large enough to take double the amount of mussels you have. Add the onion and garlic and fry gently for 5 minutes, taking care not to let them burn. Add the bay leaves, mussels, white wine, 150ml/5fl oz/scant ⅔ cup water and nutmeg. Bring to the boil, then turn the heat down, put the lid on the pan and simmer for 4 minutes, shaking the pan occasionally.

Stir the cream and parsley into the liquor around the mussels and serve with plenty of good chunky bread to mop it up.

FLAMING GINGERED PRAWNS

Prawns (shrimp) taste excellent when cooked with ginger, garlic, spring onions (scallions) and gin. Flaming the vapour removes the alcohol but leaves its aromatic flavourings.

> 4 tbsp extra-virgin olive oil
> 4 spring onions (scallions), finely sliced
> 575g/1lb 4oz raw prawns (shrimp), shelled, de-veined, rinsed
>   and dried
> 2 tsp finely chopped fresh root ginger
> 3 garlic cloves, peeled and crushed
> pinch of ground black pepper
> about 120ml/4fl oz/½ cup gin

Heat the oil in a large frying pan, then add the spring onions. Fry gently, stirring all the time, for 30 seconds. Add the prawns, ginger and garlic, and fry for a few minutes, stirring frequently, until the prawns are cooked. The time depends on the size of the prawns. They are ready when they have changed colour from grey to pinkish-orange. Stir in the pepper.

Pour the gin over the prawns, tilt the pan to one side and ignite the alcohol that runs down to that side by putting a lighted match (preferably a long one) to the vapours from the pan. Serve hot when the flames have died out.

Other

Here you'll find an interesting assortment of recipes containing garlic. Garlic can even be used to flavour beer and ice cream!

ROAST OR FRIED GARLIC

Cooked garlic has a garlicky, caramel, nutty flavour with none of the pungency of raw garlic. It's also soft, so it spreads easily. It is excellent:

- stirred into mashed potatoes (see Garlicky mashed potatoes, page 53);

- added to tomato soup, cooked rice or pasta, dips and salad dressings;

- spread on bread, or toasted bread, that you then cover with extra-virgin olive oil and sliced ripe tomatoes either raw or fried for a couple of minutes with a little olive oil, salt and pepper;

- spread over pizza dough before adding the other ingredients; or

- stirred into a white sauce intended for coating cauliflower, or into sour (soured) cream destined for baked potatoes.

   20 garlic cloves, unpeeled and with their tips snipped off with
      scissors
   25g/1oz/¼ stick butter or 2 tbsp extra-virgin olive oil

For roast garlic: preheat the oven to 180°C/350°F/gas 4. Put a piece of aluminium foil on a baking tray and put the garlic and the butter or oil into the middle. Wrap the foil over the cloves, put the baking tray in the oven and roast for 20–30 minutes, basting the garlic with the melted butter or the oil after the first 5 minutes. Remove the garlic cloves from the oven, and squeeze their soft centres into a bowl or straight into the recipe of your choice.

For fried garlic: put the cloves into a small pan with the butter and fry gently for up to 10 minutes, until tender, taking care not to let them brown. When cool enough to handle, and squeeze their soft centres into a bowl or straight into the recipe of your choice.

GARLICKY SPICED NUTS

These nuts are good as nibbles to accompany pre-dinner drinks. Use tamari soy sauce rather than the standard version because it's thicker than other soy sauces and adheres better to the nuts.

225g/8oz/1½ cups almonds
2 tbsp tamari soy sauce
1 tsp ground cumin
pinch of ground coriander
pinch of paprika
pinch of turmeric
12 garlic cloves, peeled and crushed

Preheat the oven to 180°C/350°F/gas 4.

Soak the almonds in a bowl of cold water for 30 minutes, then drain and dry on kitchen paper. Put them into a dry bowl, add the remaining ingredients and stir. Remove the nuts with a slotted spoon and put them on a baking sheet. Bake for 5 minutes, then serve warm or cold.

GARLIC BREAD

Most people love fragrant crusty garlic bread, and it's great with soup and many main courses, or even just on its own. The good news is that it's quick and easy to make. This recipe uses a French baguette.

An alternative is to make 'pulled' garlic bread. For this, you use two forks to pull out the soft crumb of an unsliced white loaf. Tear the pulled-out bread into small pieces and put them on a baking sheet. Melt the butter in a pan and stir in the garlic, then pour this over the bread and bake, uncovered, at 190°C/375°F/gas 5 for 10–15 minutes or until crisp and golden.

    1 French baguette
    6 garlic cloves, peeled and crushed
    150g/6oz/1½ sticks butter, at room temperature
    1½ tbsp chopped parsley (optional)

Preheat the oven to 180°C/350°F/gas 4.

Cut the bread into 1.5cm/½in slices, leaving them connected at the bottom.

Add the garlic to the butter and stir well. Stir in the parsley, if using.

Spread the garlic butter thickly on both sides of each slice of bread. Wrap the baguette in aluminium foil, put it on a baking tray and bake for 15–20 minutes. Serve at once.

GARLIC CROUTONS

These are good sprinkled over soups, salads, omelettes or cooked spinach. They freeze well in a sealed container. Use bread that is several days old, because fresh bread is too crumbly to cut into cubes easily.

   4 slices wholemeal (wholewheat) bread, cut into
      1cm/½in cubes
   4 tbsp extra-virgin olive oil
   4 garlic cloves, peeled and crushed

Preheat the oven to 180°C/350°F/gas 4.

Put the bread cubes into a bowl, add the olive oil and garlic and stir well. Spread them evenly on a baking sheet and bake for 15 minutes or until crisp. Use at once with hot food or allow to cool if adding to cold food.

GARLIC BREADCRUMBS

Sprinkling these crispy aromatic crumbs over soup, fried fish, or cooked spinach or tomatoes makes them taste amazing.

   3 tbsp extra-virgin olive oil or goose fat
   2 garlic cloves, peeled and crushed
   4 slices fresh brown or wholemeal (wholewheat) bread, made
      into breadcrumbs
   2 tbsp finely chopped parsley

Put the oil or goose fat into a frying pan, add the garlic and fry gently, stirring, for 2 minutes. Stir in the breadcrumbs and continue frying and stirring until the garlic breadcrumbs are crisp and golden brown. Stir in the parsley and serve hot. Alternatively, freeze in an airtight freezer bag or other container. Remove from the freezer 2 hours before you need them. Pre-heat the oven to 180°C/350°F/gas 4; then 7 minutes before you need the breadcrumbs, put them on a baking tray and bake to heat and crisp them up.

GARLIC VINEGAR

This tastes good in salad dressings, soups and casseroles.

3 large garlic cloves, peeled
450ml/16fl oz/scant 2 cups apple cider vinegar

Crush the cloves and put them into a medium-sized bowl.

Put half the vinegar into a small pan and bring to the boil, then pour it over the garlic. Leave the mixture to cool, then add the remaining vinegar. Pour the mixture into a sterilized bottle.

Leave the bottle to stand for 2 weeks, shaking it daily, then strain the vinegar and pour it into another sterilized bottle. You can eat the vinegar-preserved cloves that are left behind.

GARLIC FUDGE

Garlic may seem an unlikely flavour for fudge, but the combination of its sweetness and its typical garlic notes could give you a pleasant surprise! If you find the garlic flavour too strong, use roasted garlic cloves instead of raw ones, as these taste more mellow.

Fudge is easy to make if you:

- choose a heavy-based pan so the mixture will not burn;

- make sure the pan is large and deep, because the mixture will bubble up high;

- heat the ingredients very gently at first, because too much heat before the sugar has dissolved will make it crystallize out;

- wait until every grain of the sugar has completely dissolved before you stir the mixture;

- stir constantly when the mixture is at a 'rolling boil' (when the bubbles are large and quite slow to break);

- once you have taken the pan off the heat, wait for the mixture to cool a little before beating it, because premature beating could prevent the fudge setting; and

- leave the fudge to set at room temperature.

115g/4oz/1 stick butter

6 garlic cloves, peeled then halved lengthways

450g/1lb/2 cups granulated sugar

340g/12oz tinned (canned) evaporated milk

4 tbsp full-fat milk

Oil a deep 23cm/9in square baking tin or one of comparable size. Stand a bowl of very cold water by the hob and put a small container nearby to receive the garlic.

Put all the ingredients into a large, heavy-based pan and heat very gently until the sugar has dissolved. Remove the garlic.

Increase the heat slightly until the mixture comes to a rolling boil. Continue heating, stirring constantly, for 25–30 minutes or until the mixture reaches the 'soft-ball' stage. If you have a sugar thermometer, this means boiling until the temperature reaches 116°C/240°F. Alternatively, test by dropping a teaspoonful of the mixture into a bowl of very cold water to see if it forms a soft ball that holds its shape.

When the fudge reaches the soft-ball stage, remove the pan from the heat and leave it to stand for at least 5 minutes or until its temperature falls to 110°C/230°F. Then beat the mixture for about 10 minutes or until it loses its gloss and starts to thicken and pull away from the sides of the pan. Beating gives fudge its characteristic grainy texture.

Pour into the baking tin and leave to set at room temperature. This will take several hours – longer in warm weather, shorter in cool.

Cut the fudge into squares, remove from the tin and store in an airtight container.

CHAPTER 5

Natural Remedies

Garlic has long been prized as an aid to health and a treatment for a variety of ailments. Both raw and cooked garlic can be useful, depending on what's wrong.

How you prepare the garlic influences the amounts and proportions of its bioactive compounds (see Chapter 2).

Some people chew a fresh raw clove each day, though the release of sulfenic acid and allicin when chewing is fairly bracing! Other people add raw garlic to foods such as salad dressings (see page 61) or bruschetta (see page 48). You could drink hot water to which you have added a crushed clove, 1–2 teaspoons of honey and a squeeze of lemon juice.

How you cook garlic is important, too (see page 31).

Garlic supplements also vary in the amounts and proportions of their bioactive ingredients (see page 22). For recipes for garlic oil-macerate and garlic syrup, see pages 37 and 40 respectively.

What to Choose

This table summarizes the bioactivity of garlic's sulfur compounds:

Bioactivity	Water-soluble compounds	Oil-soluble compounds
Antioxidant and therefore anti-inflammatory	Yes	Yes
Cholesterol-lowering	Yes	Yes
Smooth-muscle relaxing	Yes	Yes
Anti-obesity	Yes	Yes
Anti-clotting	No	Yes
Anti-diabetic	No	Yes
Anti-microbial	No	Yes
Detoxifying	No	Yes
Immunity-enhancing	No	Yes

The nature and extent of this bioactivity depend on whether garlic is raw or cooked and how it is prepared, or on the type of supplement:

To get both water- and oil-soluble compounds, consume:

- Crushed or chopped garlic that you have left to stand for 30–60 minutes before eating it, mixing it with lemon juice or vinegar, or cooking it.

- A garlic-powder supplement with a high allicin yield.

To get mainly oil-soluble compounds, consume:

- Chopped or crushed garlic that has stood for 90 minutes before being eaten, mixed with lemon juice or vinegar, or cooked.

- A garlic-oil supplement if you particularly want diallyl disulfide and diallyl trisulfide.

- Garlic oil-macerate if you particularly want ajoene and vinyl dithiins.

Note that when garlic, garlic oil, garlic oil-macerate or garlic water (see page 41) are applied to the skin, their bioactive sulfur compounds not only act on local skin cells but are also absorbed into the tissue fluid and hence into the capillaries (tiny blood vessels) and tiny lymph vessels. They are then transported around the body.

How Much?

The World Health Organization advises that adults can promote health by taking one of the following each day:

- ½–1 medium clove of fresh garlic. Eat this with food – for example, crushed into a salad dressing; in warm water with honey; or added to other food towards the end of the cooking time. Allicin release begins on crushing or chopping garlic and peaks 90 minutes later. You get a good balance of water- and oil-soluble sulfur compounds if you leave chopped or crushed garlic to stand for 30–60 minutes before use.

- 0.4–1.2g garlic-powder product.

- 300–1,000mg garlic extract.

- 2–5mg garlic oil.

- Any garlic product supplying 2–5mg allicin.

Studies have found no adverse effects from eating 3–5 medium cloves a day. One study found no serious adverse effects from consuming up to 15 cloves a day for 3 months.

Precautions

Garlic has powerful biological effects, so if you are considering using it, note the following advice.

- Skin problems – do a patch test first by applying garlic to a small inconspicuous area and checking after several hours that it has not caused any irritation. Do not apply again if it has. Garlic oil lacks garlic's irritating agents (sulfenic acids and allicin) but also lacks the bioactivity of allicin and its derivatives. Be very wary of applying garlic to a child's skin.

- Vaginal or rectum/anal problems – do not use garlic locally, as it could irritate or burn.

- Stomach or digestive problems – note that large amounts of garlic can irritate the stomach and intestine.

- Bleeding disorders – note that garlic can encourage bleeding. This effect can be exaggerated by also consuming any other herb or supplement that slows blood-clotting, including fish oil, vitamin E, angelica, cloves, ginger, ginkgo, red clover, turmeric and willow.

- Pregnancy – note that normal dietary amounts of garlic are likely to be safe for the baby, but it is wise to avoid large amounts and not to apply garlic to your skin. If you are due to give birth within 2 weeks, large intakes of garlic might encourage bleeding during childbirth or associated surgical procedures.

- Breastfeeding (nursing) – avoid consuming or applying large amounts of garlic, because there are insufficient data to confirm their safety for the baby. Babies spend longer breastfeeding after their mothers have eaten garlic, probably because they like garlic-scented breast milk.

- Awaiting surgery – avoid garlic for 2 weeks before scheduled surgery, because it can prolong bleeding.

- Chronic heavy drinking – avoid consuming large amounts of garlic, because this could slow the breakdown of the liver's P450 2E1 enzyme, which helps to break down alcohol.

- Taking oral contraception ('the Pill') containing estrogen – note that garlic could speed its breakdown and endanger birth control. If you consume a lot of garlic, consider using additional birth control (such as a condom).

- Taking ciclosporine (an immunity-suppressor) – note that allicin-containing garlic products can decrease its efficacy.

- Taking medications affected by cytochrome P450 enzymes, such as paracetamol (acetaminophen); calcium-channel blockers for high blood presssure (such as nicardipine), losartan (for high blood pressure), certain anti-cancer drugs (such as paclitaxel), certain anti-fungals (such as ketoconazole), cortisol and other glucocorticoids (for allergy and autoimmune disease), chlorzoxazone (a muscle-relaxant), theophylline (for certain respiratory disorders), fentanyl (a pain-reliever), midazolam (for epilepsy), lidocaine (a local anaesthetic and a heart medication) and certain anaesthetics (such as halothane) – note that garlic can slow the breakdown of these medications, so increasing their effects. Discuss with your doctor whether to avoid or cut back on garlic.

- Taking high-blood-pressure medication with a calcium-channel blocker (such as verapamil) – note that garlic's mild blood-pressure-lowering effects might increase their action. Be sure to have regular blood-pressure checks.

- Taking anti-clotting medication (such as aspirin and warfarin) – note that garlic could further reduce clotting, encouraging bruising and bleeding, though small amounts of garlic are unlikely to be a problem. If you are on warfarin, be sure to have regular blood tests.

- Taking blood-sugar-lowering medication – note that garlic may further lower blood sugar, though normal amounts of garlic are unlikely to be a problem.

- Taking the anti-TB drug isoniazid – note that you should avoid garlic, because it could reduce the drug's absorption.

- Taking HIV/AIDS medications called non-nucleoside reverse transcriptase inhibitors (such as nevirapine); also, saquinavir as your only protease inhibitor – discuss with your doctor whether to avoid garlic.

Adverse Reactions

Garlic's oil-soluble sulfur compounds can cause the following:

- Burning mouth, heartburn, nausea, vomiting, wind, diarrhoea and appetite loss after consuming raw garlic or garlic oil on an empty stomach.

- Faintness, flushing, headache, dizziness, sweating, rapid pulse and insomnia.

- Redness, burning and blisters from prolonged use on the skin.

- Haemolytic anaemia after eating a large amount of raw garlic.

In addition, garlic can cause allergic reactions such as allergic contact dermatitis, allergic rhinitis ('hay fever'), asthma and anaphylaxis (rare but potentially fatal mouth and throat swelling, breathing difficulty and shock, which require urgent treatment with medically prescribed adrenaline). Allergic reactions are most likely in those people who work with garlic. Diallyl disulfide is often to blame because it penetrates most protective gloves. Another potential culprit is alliinase. Cross-sensitivity to other alliums or to Liliaceae plants (such as lilies, ginger and bananas) may also occur.

Ailments and Remedies

Scientists have investigated garlic more than almost any other medicinal plant, but their studies have involved many different garlic preparations or supplements, in many different doses. Also, the numbers of volunteers involved in such trials are often small. So for most disorders it is not possible to say for sure whether garlic helps or, if it does, what preparation or supplement, at what dose, is best.

To learn more about any of the studies mentioned here, enter keywords and the journal's name and year of publication into an internet search engine.

The actions I suggest should not take the place of a proper medical diagnosis and therapy. If in any doubt, see your doctor.

Acne

Skin needs adequate dietary sulfur to remain healthy, and many people are sulfur-deficient. Garlic's sulfur compounds might help. Also, its antioxidants reduce inflammation, and its sulfur compounds may kill acne bacteria.

Action: Do a patch test (see page 87).

Rub affected skin with the cut surface of a garlic clove twice a day. Alternatively, bathe the area with garlic water (see page 41) twice a day.

Include garlic in your daily diet or take a garlic-powder supplement. You need water- and oil-soluble sulfur compounds (see page 85).

Age-related cognitive decline

Garlic's antioxidants discourage memory loss and other brainpower decline by helping prevent oxidation of fatty acids, hormones and certain other substances in the brain. Garlic may also discourage artery disease, detoxify certain potentially damaging nerve-cell toxins, and encourage excretion of aluminium, lead and other heavy metals that can damage the brain.

Aged garlic extract increased memory and learning ability in mice prone to early ageing. It also discouraged degeneration in the brain's frontal lobes. Nerve cells grew better too, suggesting enhanced memory.

Phytotherapy Research, 1996

Action: Include garlic in your daily diet or take a garlic supplement. You need water- and oil-soluble sulfur compounds (see page 85).

Alzheimer's disease

Possible culprits include inflammation that encourages oxidation of brain fats, and high levels of the amino acid homocysteine. A lack of B vitamins raises homocysteine, and sufferers are particularly likely to go short of this vitamin. Garlic's anti-inflammatory antioxidants and B vitamins may help.

In Alzheimer's-prone mice, aged garlic extract helped prevent early memory loss.

Phytotherapy Research, 2007

Action: Include garlic in your daily diet or take a garlic supplement. You need water- and oil-soluble sulfur compounds (see page 85).

Artery disease

Atherosclerosis is a condition characterized by narrowing of the arteries by fatty atheroma plus stiffening of their walls by inflammation-induced scarring and calcium deposition. It is encouraged by smoking, diabetes and high blood pressure, cholesterol and trialglycerol blood fats, and an unhealthy diet and lifestyle factors that promote inflammation. At worst, a patch of atheroma ruptures, triggering a clot or bleed that causes a stroke or heart attack.

Atherosclerosis can also cause poor circulation, encouraging thin dry skin, cold feet, leg pain on walking, impotence and dementia.

Garlic is a traditional remedy; indeed:

A research review at Liverpool John Moores University suggests that the more garlic that's eaten, the less likely is artery disease to progress.

Journal of Nutrition, 2006

Scientists believe that garlic may have protective effects because various water- and oil-soluble sulfur compounds are anti-inflammatory and also boost hydrogen sulfide and inhibit ACE (see page 93) – which reduces blood pressure by expanding arteries.

In addition, they think that garlic's:

- allicin derivatives produce nitric oxide, which reduces blood pressure by relaxing smooth muscle in artery walls; they also help to counter atheroma;

- gamma-glutamyl cysteines act like ACE- (angiotensin-converting enzyme) inhibitors, a family of drugs used for high blood pressure, heart failure and strokes;

- antioxidants discourage oxidation of LDL cholesterol, and inflammation;

- manganese aids certain antioxidant enzymes and boosts HDL cholesterol (the protective type); and

- S-allyl cysteine acts like a statin (a drug used to combat high cholesterol); and its Vitamin B6 lowers levels of the amino acid homocysteine (which can damage artery walls).

Garlic has antioxidant and blood-pressure-reducing effects. It may have modest anti-clotting and cholesterol- and trialglycerol-reducing effects, too. It may also help ageing arteries remain stretchy. For example:

An Indian study reports that garlic given to mice on a fatty diet reduced blood cholesterol. Garlic also acted like statin drugs in that it blocked the enzyme (hydroxyl-methyl-glutaryl Co-A reductase) necessary for cholesterol production in the liver.

British Journal of Nutrition, 2009

An Iranian study found that garlic extract strongly inhibited angiotensin-converting enzyme (ACE) production. ACE-inhibition is known to lower blood pressure by reducing angiotensin II and bradykinin. It also reduces extra-cellular fluid by diminishing secretion of the hormone aldosterone. All this would reduce high blood pressure and so help to prevent heart failure.

Pathophysiology, 2007

Giving garlic extract to volunteers with arteriosclerosis (stiffened arteries) for 6 months reduced oxidation in their blood. Garlic boiled for 20 minutes had the same effect as raw garlic.

Life Sciences, 2006

Action: Include garlic in your daily diet or take a garlic supplement. You need water- and oil-soluble sulfur compounds (see page 85).

Arthritis

Early evidence suggests that garlic's anti-inflammatory antioxidants benefit arthritic joints.

A UK study of more than 1,000 women found osteoarthritis of the hip was less likely in those whose diet was high in garlic and other alliums. Also, in the test tube, diallyl disulphide reduced levels of cartilage-damaging enzymes.

BMC Musculoskeletal Disorders, 2010

Action: Include garlic in your daily diet or take a garlic supplement. You need both water- and oil-soluble sulfur compounds (see page 85).

Asthma

Garlic is a traditional remedy for asthma, and early evidence suggests that its anti-inflammatory antioxidants (such as quercetin) may help. It may also help in other ways:

Allicin-containing garlic extract relaxed smooth muscle in rats' windpipes. Aspirin and indomethacin, which inhibit the production of certain prostaglandins (hormone-like substances), reduced this relaxation. The conclusion was that garlic extract relaxed smooth muscle by stimulating the release of these prostaglandins.

Pharmacognosy Magazine, 2011

A study in Iran reports that giving aged garlic extract to mice with allergic airway inflammation decreased inflammation around the airways and blood vessels. It also decreased eosinophil white cells and immunoglobulin-1 antibodies, which are biochemical markers of allergy.

Iranian Journal of Allergy, Asthma and Immunology, 2008

Action: Include fresh garlic in your daily diet or take a garlic supplement. You need water- and oil-soluble sulfur compounds (see page 85).

Athlete's foot

Garlic is an anti-fungal agent, and several studies have found that garlic, or ajoene alone, is useful. For example:

A study of 50 people with athlete's foot, in New Jersey, compared one week's twice-daily applications of a 1 percent ajoene solution or the anti-fungal medication terbinafine. Garlic had a 100 percent cure rate, terbinafine 94 percent.

Journal of the American Academy of Dermatology, 2000

Action: Do a patch test (see page 87).

As ajoene cream and gel are not available commercially, apply garlic oil-macerate or garlic oil with a cotton-wool (cotton) ball twice a day. Maximize the content of allicin derivatives in homemade garlic oil-macerate by leaving newly crushed garlic to stand for 90 minutes before adding oil.

Alternatively, bathe the infected area with garlic water (see page 41).

Include garlic in your daily diet or take a garlic supplement. You need oil-soluble sulfur compounds and, in particular, ajoene (see page 13).

Bronchitis and pneumonia

Test-tube and animal studies reveal anti-inflammatory, detoxify-ing, immunity-stimulating and anti-infective properties for garlic sulfur compounds excreted through the lungs. They also show that certain garlic ingredients have the potential to break down bacterial biofilms, and to relax smooth muscle in airway walls – which would expand them and so increase air-flow.

Garlic syrup is an expectorant (encourages coughing-up of phlegm).

Garlic is also a traditional remedy for pneumonia, and studies suggest it can help viral pneumonia.

It isn't yet certain if garlic is useful for bronchitis and pneumonia, but it is worth a try.

Action: Take 1–3 teaspoons garlic syrup three times a day to help you cough up phlegm.

Alternatively, include garlic in your daily diet or take a garlic supplement. Note that you need oil-soluble sulfur compounds (see page 85).

Further options are: crush several garlic cloves, wait 30 minutes, then inhale the vapour from up to 20cm/8in away; repeat several times a day. Any initial stinging in the nose should quickly abate; if not, or if it is excessive, inhale from further away or take garlic another way.

Alternatively, do a patch test (see page 87). Rub garlic oil over your chest.

Cancer

Garlic is a traditional remedy, and preliminary studies suggest it reduces the risk of several cancers, especially those of the mouth, gullet, stomach and bowel.

Test-tube studies suggest it could help prevent or treat cancer by:

- discouraging oxidation and chronic inflammation;
- enhancing immunity;
- killing bacteria and viruses;
- influencing certain hormones;

- enhancing DNA repair;
- detoxifying certain cancer-causing agents, blocking their formation, or halting their activation; and
- reducing cancer-cell multiplication, helping to prevent them becoming invasive, or promoting their suicide (apoptosis).

For example:

A test-tube study of the effects of 34 vegetable extracts on 8 types of cancer-cell found that garlic was by far the strongest inhibitor of their multiplication. It didn't inhibit the multiplication of normal cells.

Food Chemistry, 2009

A German study found that steeping raw meat in a garlicky marinade greatly reduced the content of cancer-encouraging heterocyclic amines in the cooked meat.

Journal of Agricultural and Food Chemistry, 2007

Test-tube research found that a garlic lectin (sugar-binding protein) strongly reduced cancer-cell multiplication and induced apoptosis.

Food Research International, 2001

However, studies in people paint a much less rosy picture – as, for example, in the following review (although the number of studies good enough to be selected for the review was relatively small, as were the numbers of people studied):

A review of 19 selected trials in 1955–2007 found no credible evidence for a relation between garlic intake and a reduced risk of breast, lung, stomach or womb cancer. Also, only very limited evidence supported a relation between garlic intake and a reduced risk of colon, gullet, kidney, larynx, mouth, ovary or prostate cancer.

American Journal of Clinical Nutrition, 2009

Action: Hedge your bets by including garlic in your daily diet or taking a garlic supplement. You need water– and oil-soluble sulfur compounds (see page 85).

Cold sores

In the test tube, at least, *Herpes simplex virus* type 1, which causes cold sores, is sensitive to allicin and its derivatives, in particular ajoene.

Action: Do a patch test (see page 87).

Smear a little petroleum jelly ('Vaseline') on to the skin around the sore, then apply a sliver cut from a garlic clove and leave it for as long as it will stay there; repeat twice a day.

Alternatively, apply the oil from a garlic oil-macerate to the sore several times a day. These methods also exclude air from the sore, which is helpful.

Another option is to bathe the infected area with garlic water (see page 41).

A final option is to apply allicin cream. Any stinging and smell soon go.

In addition, include garlic in your diet or take a garlic supplement. You need oil-soluble sulfur compounds (see page 85).

Colds, coughs, sore throats, sinusitis and 'flu

Garlic is a traditional remedy. Any success is probably because of its anti-microbial, anti-inflammatory and immunity-enhancing compounds. For example, test-tube studies show that *Parainfluenza virus* type 3 and *Human rhinovirus* type 2 are sensitive to garlic.

This study suggests that garlic helps to prevent and treat colds:

146 volunteers took either an allicin-containing garlic supplement or a placebo (dummy medication) for 12 weeks in winter. Those taking garlic had only 24 colds while those who took the placebo had 65; also, those [colds] they had were shorter and their chances of re-infection were reduced.

Advances in Therapy, 2001

Action: Take garlic in honey, because garlic is powerfully antiseptic, while honey is soothing and healing. To do this, crush 10 garlic cloves, then leave to stand for 10–90 minutes before stirring the garlic into a 450g/1lb jar of clear honey. Take 1 teaspoon every 2 hours.

Alternatively, take a teaspoon of garlic syrup (see page 40) every 2 hours.

Alternatively, crush several garlic cloves, then wait for 30 minutes before inhaling the fumes from up to 20cm/8in away. Repeat several times a day. Any initial stinging in the nose should quickly abate, but if not, or if it is excessive, inhale from further away or take garlic in another form.

Alternatively, take a garlic supplement. You need oil-soluble sulfur compounds (see page 85).

Alternatively, take a pure-allicin supplement.

Take a warm garlic bath (see page 41).

For a sore throat, gargle with garlic water (see page 41).

Cramps

Research suggests that garlic can help tense smooth-muscle cells to relax (see 'Asthma'). So it might also help period pain or intestinal colic.

Action: Include garlic in your daily diet or take a garlic supplement. You need both water- and oil-soluble sulfur compounds (see page 85).

Cystitis

Those of garlic's anti-inflammatory and anti-microbial agents that make it to the bladder may help to counter a urine infection. Also, it is possible, though unproven, that garlic's smooth-muscle-relaxing properties might help to relax cystitis-like symptoms caused by unusually tense smooth muscle in the bladder wall.

Action: Include garlic in your daily diet or take a garlic supplement. You need water- and oil-soluble sulfur compounds (see page 85).

Dandruff

Scalp flaking is often associated with infection with the fungus *Malassezia furfur*. Garlic's anti-fungal activity means it might be effective.

Action: Do a patch test (see page 87).

Apply garlic water (see page 41) to your scalp, cover with a towel for 1 hour, then rinse off the bits of garlic before shampooing. Repeat once or twice a week.

Alternatively, mix 2 crushed cloves of garlic with a tablespoon of coconut oil. Use the mixture to massage your scalp for 5 minutes, then cover with a hot towel for 20 minutes before shampooing.

Alternatively, massage your scalp with garlic oil, then continue as above.

Alternatively, use a garlic shampoo and conditioner (available on the internet).

Include garlic in your daily diet or take a garlic supplement. You need water- and oil-soluble sulfur compounds (see page 85).

Diabetes

Many studies show that raw garlic reduces blood sugar in animals with type-2 diabetes (the common sort). Researchers attribute this to allicin and its derivatives. For example, garlic oil and diallyl trisulfide improved blood sugar in diabetic rats by increasing insulin release and reducing insulin resistance:

In an Indian study, rats were given a diet of 65 percent fruit sugar (which induces type-2-diabetes); or 65 percent fruit sugar and raw garlic; or a 'control' diet of 65 percent cornstarch [cornflour]. After 8 weeks, the fruit-sugar group had higher blood sugar, insulin and insulin resistance than the controls, but the gains were lower in those that had consumed garlic.

Nutrition, Metabolism and Cardiovascular Diseases, 2011

It is not yet known whether garlic helps to prevent or treat diabetes in humans, but research suggests it might help to prevent diabetes-associated heart disease, which is responsible for most deaths in people with diabetes.

Action: Until we know more, include garlic in your daily diet or take a garlic supplement. You need oil-soluble sulfur compounds (see page 85).

Diarrhoea

Garlic's allicin and certain of its derivatives (such as diallyl disulphide) can kill bacteria such as *Escherichia coli* and salmonellae, which can cause gastroenteritis. Garlic can also help to cure diarrhoea caused by infection with the protozoon *Cryptosporidium*.

In addition, garlic can help to relieve diarrhoea associated with antibiotics, or irritable bowel syndrome, by restoring a normal balance of gut bacteria.

Action: Include garlic in your daily diet or take a garlic supplement. You need water- and oil-soluble sulfur compounds (see page 85).

Fatigue

Garlic is a traditional remedy. Early research suggests that it promotes exercise endurance. Also, garlic promotes production of hydrogen sulphide and nitric oxide, both of which relax arteries, so increasing blood flow to muscles. This enhances energy, post-exercise recovery and muscle growth.

A study in which rats did endurance exercise 5 times a week found that giving aged garlic extract 30 minutes beforehand facilitated aerobic sugar metabolism, reduced oxidation and, by widening arteries, promoted the muscles' oxygen supply.

Biological & Pharmaceutical Bulletin, 2006

Action: Include garlic in your daily diet or take a garlic supplement. You need water- and oil-soluble sulfur compounds (see page 85).

Fluid retention

Garlic is a traditional remedy in certain countries.

An Iranian study found that garlic extract strongly inhibited the formation of angiotensin-converting enzyme (ACE). ACE-inhibition is known to reduce fluid retention by diminishing secretion of the hormones aldosterone and anti-diuretic hormone.

Pathophysiology, 2007

A study in Chile found that garlic-powder capsules increased urine production in dogs. The effects were dose-dependent,

peaked within 40 minutes and fell to their initial levels within
2¹/₂ hours.

Journal of Ethnopharmacology, 1991

Action: Include garlic in your daily diet or take a garlic supplement.
You need water- and oil-soluble sulfur compounds (see page 85).

Gallstones

Garlic has been claimed to increase bile flow. If so, it would
discourage gallstones, which occur when bile stagnates in the gall-
bladder. What's more, garlic is rich in antioxidants, which, studies
suggest, discourage gallstones. Garlic may also have a cholesterol-
lowering effect in both blood and bile.

Researchers in India found that when mice on a gallstone-
promoting diet were given raw or cooked garlic, the bile's
cholesterol concentration was reduced and gallstones
discouraged. Raw garlic was the most effective.

British Journal of Nutrition, 2009

Action: Include garlic in your daily diet or take a garlic supplement.
You need water- and oil-soluble sulfur compounds (see page 85).

Hay fever

Garlic is a traditional remedy. Any success probably stems from its
anti-inflammatory and anti-histamine constituents.

Action: Eat more garlic or take a garlic supplement in the weeks before and during your usual hay-fever season. You need water- and oil-soluble sulfur compounds (see page 85).

Heart attack

Heart attacks are encouraged by atherosclerosis (see 'Artery disease', page 92), chronic infection (see 'Infection', page 111), diabetes (see page 102), high blood pressure (see page 108), a tendency to inflammation (see page 112) or blood-clotting (see below) and high cholesterol (see page 109). Garlic may help to prevent these. It has certainly been noted that people who eat a lot of garlic tend to have lower rates of coronary heart disease – though this does not, of course, constitute proof.

Test-tube studies show that garlic can decrease blood-clotting by:

- making tiny particles in blood (platelets) less sticky and less likely to clump together to form a blood clot;

- boosting nitric-oxide production (this ability is retained by heat-treated and aged garlic products);

- decreasing blood sugar (this is helpful because sugary blood is more likely to clot); or

- decreasing fibrinogen (high levels of this blood-clotting protein encourage clots; they also rise during inflammation).

A review of randomized controlled trials done between 1966 and 2000 found that garlic modestly decreased platelet clumping in the test tube.

Archives of Internal Medicine, 2001

An Argentinian study found that 6–10 minutes of boiling in water, or oven-heating, destroyed the anti-platelet-clumping ability of whole garlic and reduced that of crushed garlic. However, more than 10 minutes of either treatment destroyed this anti-clotting ability, as did microwaving. The researchers conclude that crushing garlic before cooking it for a short time helps to conserve some anti-clotting ability.

Journal of Agricultural and Food Chemistry, 2007

Garlic may also make permanent damage from a heart attack less likely:

A study at the University of Connecticut gave freshly crushed garlic, roasted garlic, or no garlic, to rats for 30 days. The blood supply to the heart was then reduced for 30 minutes. Both types but particularly the freshly crushed garlic helped prevent heart damage. This also increased certain anti-inflammatory factors, thanks to hydrogen-sulphide production.

Journal of Agricultural and Food Chemistry, 2009

In addition, garlic may discourage abnormal heart rhythm after a heart attack (or, indeed, at any other time). But while garlic does help to prevent clots in the test tube, several small studies suggest that it does not work for people; for example:

A study of 14 volunteers found little or no effect on platelet-clumping 4 hours after taking capsules of garlic oil-macerate.

Wojcikowski, 2007

Action: Until we know more, include garlic in your daily diet or take a garlic supplement. You need water- and oil-soluble sulfur compounds (see page 85).

High blood pressure

Research suggests that this traditional remedy reduces high blood pressure (defined as more than 140/90mmHg). Falls in blood pressure produced by taking garlic compare with those from common blood-pressure medications (such as beta-blockers and ACE inhibitors). For example:

In a study at the University of Adelaide, Australia, 50 volunteers with high blood pressure despite medication were put into two groups. One took aged garlic extract plus their medication for 12 weeks; the other just their medication. Those on garlic had an average fall of 10 mmHg in their systolic blood pressure (the upper of a reading's two figures).

Maturitas, 2010

A review of 10 good studies up to 2008 found that garlic reduced high systolic blood pressure by 16 mmHg and reduced diastolic blood pressure (the lower of a reading's two figures) by 9 mmHg, compared with a placebo (dummy medication).

Annals of Pharmacotherapy, 2008

The numbers of people that have been studied are relatively small. However, if garlic does indeed help, this is probably because it:

- discourages atherosclerosis (see 'Artery disease');

- contains gamma-glutamyl cysteines – natural angiotensin-converting enzyme inhibitors (ACE inhibitors) that reduce blood pressure by expanding arteries;

- releases hydrogen sulphide (from polysulfides in chopped or crushed raw garlic), which expands arteries;

- promotes nitric oxide production, which expands arteries (this ability is retained by heat-treated and aged garlic products);

- has prostaglandin-like effects, which reduce blood pressure by relaxing smooth muscle in artery walls; and

- contains substances that activate sodium-pump enzymes, which maintain low sodium levels in cells.

In addition, one small study suggests that vitamin C enhances garlic's blood-pressure-lowering effect. Also, studies suggest that this effect lasts for up to 24–48 hours.

Action: Include garlic in your daily diet or take a garlic supplement. You need water- and oil-soluble sulfur compounds (see page 85).

Eat plenty of vitamin-C-containing foods.

High cholesterol

High levels of low-density lipoprotein (LDL) cholesterol and total cholesterol, and a low level of high-density-lipoprotein (HDL) cholesterol, plus a lifestyle that encourages oxidation of LDL cholesterol, encourages heart attacks and strokes. Scientists have found that low HDL cholesterol is four times better at predicting heart attacks than high LDL cholesterol, and eight times better than high total cholesterol.

Many studies in the 1980s and early 1990s suggested that garlic might help to inhibit cholesterol production, increase cholesterol excretion and protect LDL cholesterol from oxidation.

Since then, though, high-quality studies have suggested that garlic does not help significantly. So current medical opinion is that garlic is 'possibly ineffective'.

In a US trial, 192 adults with raised total and LDL cholesterol took raw garlic, powdered garlic, aged garlic extract, or a placebo (dummy medication) 6 days a week for six months. The daily garlic dose equated to a medium-sized clove. None of the three types of garlic had significant effects on cholesterol.

Archives of Internal Medicine, 2007

However, it's just possible that certain formulations of supplement could have positive effects. For example:

In a Russian study, 42 men with mildly high cholesterol took timed-release garlic-powder tablets for 12 weeks. There was a moderate decrease in total and LDL cholesterol, and an increase in HDL cholesterol.

Journal of Atherosclerosis and Thrombosis, 2008

Action: Until we know more, include garlic in your daily diet or take a garlic supplement. You need water- and oil-soluble sulfur compounds (see page 85).

Indigestion

Garlic is a traditional remedy.

Action: Include garlic in your daily diet or take a garlic supplement. You need water- and oil-soluble sulfur compounds (see page 85), though stop if either worsens your indigestion.

Infection

Garlic has been used for millennia to treat infections. In World War II, garlic became known as 'Russian penicillin' because the new antibiotics were in short supply and Red Army physicians used garlic instead. Today, garlic remains a popular anti-infective agent worldwide. Indeed, many Russian hospitals still use the vapour of freshly chopped garlic to combat infection.

Test-tube studies show the following:

- Garlic has anti-bacterial effects against bacilli, brucellae, enterobacter, mycobacteria, pseudomonas, staphylococci, streptococci and vibro bacteria as well as *Campylobacter jejuni, Cryptococcus neoformans. Enterococcus faecalis, Escherichia coli, Helicobacter pylori, Klebsiella pneumoniae, Neisseria gonorrhoeae, Proteus vulgaris* and *Salmonella enteritidis.* Allicin-containing supplements may help to cure infections caused by the 'superbug' methicillin-resistant *Staphylococcus aureus* (MRSA). Bacteria can become resistant to antibiotics but not to garlic.

- Garlic has anti-viral effects against coxsackie viruses and human cytomegaloviruses, as well as *Herpes simplex* types 1 and 2, *Human immunodeficiency virus* type 1, *Human rhinovirus* type 2, *Influenza virus* type B, *Parainfluenza virus* type 3, *Vaccinia virus* and *Vesicular stomatitis virus*. Garlic may also enhance the efficacy of 'flu vaccine.

- Garlic has anti-fungal effects against aspergillus, microsporum and trichophyton as well as *Cryptococcus neoformans, Pneumocystis jirovecii* and various yeasts, including the yeast-like fungus *Candida albicans*. Garlic can be more potent than certain anti-fungal medications, including amphotericin B, gentian violet, griseofulvin, ketoconazole and nystatin.

- Garlic has anti-protozoal effects against cryptosporidia,
  Entamoeba histolytica, *Toxoplasma gondii* and various types of
  plasmodium (which causes malaria).

Few studies have been done in people to compare garlic with anti-biotics, anti-viral, anti-fungal or anti-protozoal drugs. However, it would seem that garlic is well worth trying along with such drugs or (for an infection that isn't serious) on its own.

Action: To help prevent or treat infection, include garlic in your daily diet or take a garlic supplement. You need oil-soluble sulfur compounds (see page 85).

Inflammation

Many garlic constituents have antioxidant or other anti-inflammatory actions. These include its flavonoids, saponins and many of its sulfur compounds. This helps to explain its reputation for helping to treat diseases that involve inflammation, such as allergy, Alzheimer's, arthritis, asthma, atherosclerosis, cancer, diabetes, eczema, hay fever, heart attacks, infection, inflammatory bowel disease, metabolic syndrome, multiple sclerosis, osteoporosis, psoriasis and strokes.

A Canadian test-tube study shows that sulfenic acid (produced from alliin by the enzyme alliinase) is the fastest antioxidant ever seen. The researchers believe this helps explain garlic's medicinal benefits.

Angewandte Chemie, 2009

A research review at the University of Texas notes that many inflammatory diseases have been linked with activation of an inflammation-inducing substance called nuclear transcription factor κB. The pathway that activates this factor can be interrupted by substances derived from various spices and herbs, as well as by diallyl sulfide, S-allylmercaptocysteine and ajoene from garlic. This, they say, 'provides reasoning for seasoning'.

Annals of the New York Academy of Sciences, 2004

However, a study in people with pro-inflammatory risk factors found that garlic had no effect on commonly measured biomarkers of inflammation:

In a study of 90 overweight smokers, taking a daily garlic-powder supplement did not reduce these biomarkers of inflammation.

American Journal of Clinical Nutrition, 2006

Action: Until we know more, include garlic in your daily diet by taking a garlic supplement. You need water- and oil-soluble sulfur compounds (see page 85).

Metabolic syndrome

This syndrome (also called pre-diabetes or syndrome X) greatly encourages diabetes, heart disease and strokes, affects one in five adults and is defined by having three of more of these factors:

- Insulin resistance.
- 'Apple-shaped' body, with fat around the waist.
- High blood pressure.
- High blood fats.

• Low HDL-cholesterol (the protective sort).

Researchers suspect that inflammation and oxidation play a part. It is certain that affected people are prone to high levels of C-reactive protein, indicating inflammation. Recent research suggests that garlic discourages metabolic syndrome:

In an Indian study, rats ate a diet of 65 percent fruit sugar (a diabetes-inducing diet), or a diet of 65 percent fruit sugar and raw garlic, or a control diet of 65 percent cornstarch (cornflour). After 8 weeks, both the fruit-sugar groups had raised blood sugar, insulin, trialglycerols, uric-acid and insulin resistance. But these gains were lower in the group that also consumed garlic. The conclusion was that garlic improves insulin sensitivity and metabolic syndrome in rats on a diabetes-inducing diet.

Nutrition, Metabolism and Cardiovascular Diseases, 2011

Action: Include garlic in your daily diet or take a garlic supplement. You need water- and oil-soluble sulfur compounds (see page 85).

Mouth ulcers

Also called aphthous ulcers or canker sores, these can be extraordinarily painful.

Action: Do a patch test (see page 87).

Dab an ulcer with the cut end of a garlic clove several times a day. But don't repeat this if the pain worsens the first time.

Include raw garlic in your daily diet or take a garlic supplement. You need water- and oil-soluble sulfur compounds (see page 85).

Nail infections

Garlic may help to treat a fungal nail infection.

Action: Do a patch test on the adjacent skin (see page 87).

Apply garlic oil (for example, from a garlic perle) to the infected nail and adjacent skin 2 or 3 times a day for 6 months for fingernails, or a year for toenails. Alternatively, use the oil from garlic oil-macerate (see page 37).

Include garlic in your daily diet or take a garlic supplement. You need water- and oil-soluble sulfur compounds (see page 85).

Neuralgia

Some people with nerve pain such as trigeminal neuralgia report that repeated applications of garlic to the painful area are helpful. Garlic might work by producing hydrogen sulfide and nitric oxide, which expand arteries, thus improving the blood supply to nerves. Garlic might also help by supplying anti-inflammatory compounds. In addition, its allixin is said to encourage nerve growth and wellbeing.

However, if pain results from pressure on a nerve, as with sciatica, garlic is unlikely to help.

Action: Do a patch test (see page 87).

Apply the garlicky oil from a garlic oil-macerate (see page 37) to the painful area several times a day. Maximize the content of allicin derivatives in homemade garlic oil-macerate by leaving the newly crushed garlic to stand for 90 minutes before adding the oil.

Include garlic in your daily diet or take a garlic supplement. You need oil-soluble sulfur compounds (see page 85).

Obesity

Garlic is reputed to aid weight loss. Early research suggests that it might help by:

- encouraging heat production by brown fat (metabolically active fat between the shoulder-blades), stimulating the breakdown of trialglycerol blood fats;

- inactivating gastric lipase, an enzyme needed for fat digestion;

- reducing appetite;

- making pre-adipocytes (fat-cell precursors) less likely to develop into adipocytes; and

- reducing the fat absorbed from a meal.

For example:

In an Indian study, rats were fed a diet of 65 percent fruit sugar (which induces type-2-diabetes), or a diet of 65 percent fruit sugar and raw garlic, or a 'control' diet of 65 percent cornstarch [cornflour]. Those given fruit sugar and garlic gained less weight over 8 weeks.

Nutrition, Metabolism and Cardiovascular Diseases, 2011

French researchers report that vinyl dithiin made pre-adipocytes less likely to accumulate fat or produce inflammatory molecules (such as interleukin-6).

Journal of Nutrition, 2009

Japanese researchers report that rats on a high-fat diet given a garlic-powder supplement for 28 days lost weight. The garlic increased their adrenaline and noradrenaline – hormones that stimulate trialglycerol metabolism and are thought to boost heat production in brown fat. Garlic also increased uncoupling protein – which similarly increases heat production in brown fat. The researchers also report that alliin, diallyl disulfide or diallyl trisulfide increased adrenaline and noradrenaline.

Journal of Nutrition, 1999

This study found that garlic's ajoenes inactivate gastric lipase, the enzyme needed for digestion of fats.

Biochimica et Biophysica Acta, 1989

Action: Until we know more, include garlic in your daily diet or take a garlic supplement. You need water- and oil-soluble sulfur compounds (see page 85).

Osteoporosis

Research suggests that inflammation and oxidation play an important part in this bone-thinning condition, in which case garlic's anti-inflammatory antioxidants might help.

Action: Until we know more, include garlic in your daily diet or take a garlic supplement. You need water- and oil-soluble sulfur compounds (see page 85).

Peptic ulcer

A peptic ulcer can develop if something interferes with the stomach's protective mucus, lining or acid. Contrary to popular belief, most people with ulcers do not make too much acid. In fact, many make too little. Inflammation caused by infection with *Helicobacter pylori* bacteria is a major cause, and these bacteria are becoming increasingly resistant to antibiotics. While garlic has anti-bacterial properties in the test tube, giving garlic to people with a peptic ulcer who are infected with these bacteria does not help. So the current thinking is that garlic may be ineffective.

Action: Until we know more, include garlic in your daily diet or take a garlic supplement, but stop if your symptoms worsen. You need water- and oil-soluble sulfur compounds (see page 85).

Piles (haemorrhoids)

Piles occur when spongy pads in the walls of the back passage enlarge. They then readily become inflamed, triggering itching, bleeding and discomfort. Possible causes include constipation and fragile veins. Garlic might help because of its anti-inflammatory compounds, fibre (which helps prevent constipation) and vitamin C and flavonoids (which strengthen veins).

Inserting garlic into the back passage is a traditional remedy that is best avoided as it can irritate or burn.

Action: Include garlic in your daily diet or take a garlic supplement. You need water- and oil-soluble sulfur compounds (see page 85).

Poor circulation

Garlic is known as a 'warming' herb because it expands arteries, so boosting circulation. It may also help to prevent or treat artery disease. It also makes blood less sticky, which aids blood flow.

Action: Include garlic in your daily diet or take a garlic supplement. You need water- and oil-soluble sulfur compounds (see page 85).

Poor immunity

Early studies confirm the common belief that garlic boosts immunity, showing, for example, that it influences several sorts of white cell by:

- stimulating the ability of natural killer cells to destroy virus-infected and cancer cells;
- increasing the activity of macrophages (which engulf foreign bacteria);
- activating helper-T cells (which encourage the growth and activation of cytotoxic or 'cell-killer' T cells);
- maximizing the bactericidal activity of macrophages; and
- influencing the sorts of antibodies produced by B cells.

Action: Include garlic in your daily diet or take a garlic supplement. You need oil-soluble sulfur compounds (see page 85).

Premature ageing and death

Garlic's vitamin C and other antioxidants help to counter early ageing of skin, joints and arteries and reduce inflammation associated with heart disease, arthritis and Alzheimer's. Garlic may also discourage certain cancers and strokes. Finally, pectin in the garlic-clove skin helps to eliminate from the body heavy metals such as aluminium and lead, which encourage cells to age prematurely.

In mice prone to early aging, aged garlic extract increased lifespan.

Phytotherapy Research, 1996

Action: Include garlic in your daily diet or take a garlic supplement. You need water- and oil-soluble sulfur compounds (see page 85).

Prostate enlargement

Preliminary evidence suggests that garlic might improve urine flow and make urination less frequent in men with benign prostate enlargement.

Action: Until we know more, include garlic in your daily diet or by taking a garlic supplement. You need water- and oil-soluble sulfur compounds (see page 85).

Psoriasis

This condition causes patches of thick flaking skin overlying inflammation on the knees, elbows, scalp or elsewhere.

Garlic's anti-inflammatory constituents may soothe the inflammation.

Action: Do a patch test (see page 87).

Apply garlicky oil from a garlic oil-macerate (see page 37), or garlic oil (for example, from a garlic 'perle'), to affected areas twice a day. Maximize the content of allicin derivatives in homemade garlic oil-macerate by standing the newly crushed garlic for 90 minutes before adding the oil.

Alternatively, bathe infected areas with garlic water (see page 41).

Include garlic in your daily diet or take a garlic supplement. You need water- and oil-soluble sulfur compounds (see page 85).

Ringworm

This results from a fungal skin infection. There is good evidence that garlic and, in particular, ajoene, can help:

In a Venezuelan study, 60 soldiers with ringworm or 'jock itch' were treated with ajoene gel, or cream containing terbinafine (an anti-fungal drug), for 2 months. Healing occurred in 73 and 71 percent of the two groups respectively. The researchers concluded that ajoene is useful.

*Arzneimittel-Forschung,*1999

Action: Do a patch test (see page 87).

Since ajoene gel isn't available commercially, apply garlic oil-macerate twice a day until 14 days after the skin has healed. Maximize the content of allicin derivatives in homemade garlic oil-macerate by leaving the newly crushed garlic to stand for 90 minutes before adding the oil.

Alternatively, bathe the infected area with garlic water (see page 41).

Include garlic in your daily diet or take a garlic supplement. You need oil-soluble sulfur compounds (see page 85).

Sex problems

Scientific evidence now backs up the belief that garlic increases libido and discourages impotence. For example, nitric oxide is now known to be vital for penile erection, and garlic increases nitric-oxide levels. Garlic also expands arteries, improving blood flow to the hormone-producing glands and the genitals. What's more, garlic boosts testosterone, and garlic's diallyl disulfide boosts luteinizing hormone (a pituitary hormone that regulates testosterone production).

Japanese researchers found that rats fed with garlic had higher testosterone and lower corticosterone after 28 days. Also, giving diallyl disulfide increased luteinizing hormone.

Journal of Nutrition, 2001

Action: Include garlic in your daily diet or take a garlic supplement. You need water- and oil-soluble sulfur compounds (see page 85).

Shingles

Folk wisdom has it that applying garlic reduces the pain and itching of this varicella-zoster viral infection. After chickenpox (usually contracted many years before), these viruses lie dormant in the sensory nerve cells of a particular nerve until some kind of trigger reawakens them to cause shingles in the area supplied by that nerve.

Garlic inactivates the related viruses *Herpes simplex* 1 and 2. While I can find no mention of garlic acting against varicella-zoster viruses, it must be worth a try.

Action: Do a patch test (see page 87).

Apply garlic oil from a garlic perle, or the garlicky oil from a garlic oil-macerate (see page 37), twice a day. Maximize the content of allicin derivatives in homemade garlic oil-macerate by leaving the newly crushed garlic to stand for 90 minutes before adding the oil.

Alternatively, bathe the infected area with garlic water (see page 41).

Include garlic in your daily diet or take a garlic supplement. You need oil-soluble sulfur compounds (see page 85).

Skin infections

Garlic is a useful treatment for bacterial, viral and fungal skin infections. In World War I, the British Government paid a shilling a pound for garlic to prevent wound infections.

Action: Do a patch test (see page 87).

Apply garlic oil from a garlic perle, or the oily part of a garlic oil-macerate (see page 37), twice a day. Maximize the content of allicin derivatives in homemade garlic oil-macerate by leaving the newly crushed garlic to stand for 90 minutes before adding the oil.

Alternatively, bathe the infected area with garlic water (see page 41).

Include garlic in your daily diet or take a garlic supplement. You need oil-soluble sulfur compounds (see page 85).

Strokes

Most strokes ('brain attacks') are thrombotic (resulting from a clot in a brain artery); the rest are haemorrhagic (resulting from bleeding from a brain artery).

Strokes are encouraged by atherosclerosis (see 'Artery disease', page 92), chronic infection (see page 111), diabetes (see page 102), high blood pressure (see page 108), an increased tendency to inflammation (see page 112) or blood-clotting (see 'Heart attacks', page 106), and high cholesterol (see page 109). Garlic may help to prevent these.

Action: Include garlic in your daily diet or take a garlic supplement. You need water- and oil-soluble sulfur compounds (see page 85).

Thrush

Garlic is a useful remedy for infection of the mouth or skin with the yeast-like fungus *Candida albicans*. Test-tube studies show garlic's allicin is highly effective and ajoene inhibits the fungal growth.

Action: Include garlic in your daily diet or take a garlic supplement. You need oil-soluble sulfur compounds (see page 85).

If you have a mouth infection, chew then spit out a raw garlic clove several times a day, though stop if this causes irritation.

If you have a skin infection, first do a patch test (see page 87). If satisfactory, apply garlic oil (for example, from a garlic perle or garlic oil-macerate) several times a day.

Alternatively, bathe the infected area with garlic water (see page 31).

In the case of a vaginal infection, take garlic as above but do not be tempted to follow the sometimes-given advice to insert a raw garlic clove in the vagina because it could become stuck, in which case it could encourage other infection.

Toothache

This results from bacterial decay exposing nerve endings in a tooth's dentine. Garlic is a traditional remedy and its success may be because it kills infecting bacteria, or reduces inflammation.

Action: Apply crushed garlic that you have left to stand for 90 minutes, or garlic oil (for example, from a garlic perle or garlic oil-macerate – see page 37). Limit the first application to 10 minutes and stop if it irritates your gums. Repeat four times a day.

Alternatively, rinse your mouth with garlic water (see page 41) four times a day.

Include garlic in your daily diet or take a garlic supplement. You need oil-soluble sulfur compounds (see page 85).

Warts and verrucas

Garlic's anti-viral effects are a good enough reason to try it for warts and verrucas. Several studies now provide backing:

In a study of 28 people, warts vanished within 1–2 weeks in those who applied an oil-soluble garlic extract twice a day.

International Journal of Dermatology, 2005

In this study warts on the hands of five children were treated with garlic. Each night, a clove's cut surface was rubbed over each wart, any stray juice cleaned from the surrounding area, and the wart covered overnight with a sticking plaster (adhesive bandage). All the warts disappeared within 7–12 weeks. The treatment was well tolerated apart from in one child, who had itching.

Pediatric Dermatology, 2002

Action: Do a patch test (see page 87).

Smear a little petroleum jelly ('Vaseline') on to the skin around the wart. Apply to the wart either crushed raw garlic that has been left to stand for 90 minutes, garlic oil from a garlic perle or the garlicky oil from a garlic oil-macerate (see page 37). Maximize the content of allicin derivatives in homemade garlic oil-macerate by standing the newly crushed garlic for 90 minutes before adding the oil. Cover with a large sticking plaster or piece of duct tape, and repeat each day until the wart goes (probably 7–10 days, though it may take several weeks to disappear).

Include garlic in your daily diet or take a garlic supplement. You need oil-soluble sulfur compounds (see page 85).

Useful Addresses and Websites

Below you'll find a selection of companies and organizations concerned with garlic. Farmers' markets are often a good source of the more unusual varieties of garlic and you can find their details from your local council or library, or on the internet. Some garlic-growing countries have festivals to celebrate the garlic harvest; you can find information about these on the internet too.

UK

Ecospray Limited
Tel: 0044 1760 756100
www.ecospray.com
This company makes ECOguard liquid or granules, a garlic concentrate that deters slugs and snails.

The Garlic Farm
Tel: 0044 1983 865378
www.thegarlicfarm.co.uk
This farm, on the Isle of Wight, grows garlic, sells garlic and garlic products and mounts a Garlic Festival each summer.

The Garlic Information Centre

Tel: 0044 1424 892440

This offers information about garlic's health benefits.

Canada

Boundary Garlic Farm

Tel: 001 250 449 2152

www.garlicfarm.ca/

This company in British Columbia sells garlic for planting and offers information about growing garlic.

US

The Garlic Store

Tel: 001 970 223 0028

www.thegarlicstore.com/

The Garlic Store in Colorado sells garlic for planting as well as garlic braids, garlic oil, vinegar and other food products, and items such as garlic presses, peelers and keepers.

The Gilroy Garlic Festival

Tel: 001 408 842 1625

www.gilroygarlicfestival.com

This annual festival is held in Gilroy, California.

Gourmet Garlic Gardens

Tel: 001 325 348 3049

www.gourmetgarlicgardens.com

This company offers information about garlic and offers garlic and garlic products directly from market gardeners – just like at a local farmers' market.

Australia

Rochford Organic Garlic

Tel: 0061 2 6736 3062

www.rochfordorganicgarlic.com.au

This company in New South Wales sells garlic, including purple garlic and elephant garlic. It welcomes group visits by arrangement and offers a consultation service for new growers. It also has a limited supply of oriental purple seed garlic available for sale each year.

Index